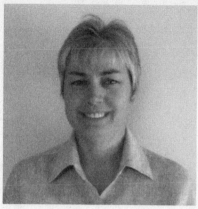

Jennifer Kelly has degrees in Nursing, Women's Studies and Education (Adult) from Charles Darwin University and Deakin University, Australia. She is a Registered Nurse and Midwife. She has worked for many years in the area of women's health in a variety of roles and locations throughout Australia. Jennifer has a wide range of teaching and research experiences that include nursing, health promotion and Women's Studies. She lives with her partner by the ocean on the Surf Coast of Victoria, Australia.

Zest for Life

LESBIANS' EXPERIENCES OF MENOPAUSE

JENNIFER KELLY

Spinifex Press Pty Ltd
504 Queensberry Street
North Melbourne, Vic. 3051
Australia
women@spinifexpress.com.au
http://www.spinifexpress.com.au

First published 2005
Copyright © Jennifer Kelly
Copyright on layout, Spinifex Press, 2005

This book is copyright. Apart from any fair dealings for the purpose of private study, research, criticism or review, as permitted under the Copyright Act, this book may not be reproduced in whole or in part by any process, stored in or introduced into a retrieval system or transmitted, in any form or by any means (electronic, mechanical, photocopying, recording or otherwise), without prior written permission of the copyright owner and the above publisher of the book.

Copyright for educational purposes
Where copies of part or the whole book are made under part VB of the Copyright Act, the law requires the prescribed procedures be followed. For information, contact the Copyright Agency Limited.

Edited and indexed by Kerry Biram
Cover design by Deb Snibson
Typeset by Claire Warren
Printed and bound by McPherson's Printing Group

National Library of Australia
cataloguing-in-publication data:

Kelly, Jennifer.
    Zest for life : lesbians' experiences of menopause.

    Bibliography.
    Includes index.
    ISBN 1 876756 46 2.

    1. Menopause. 2. Lesbians. 3. Body image in women.
    I. Title.

612.665

For lesbians everywhere . . .

JK

Contents

Preface

My reasons for writing this book are twofold. Firstly, I wanted to give something back to the many lesbians who freely shared their thoughts and experiences with me, a total stranger. Lesbians, like members of other oppressed groups, have for too long been giving their/our information to academics, researchers and bureaucrats with little, if any, feedback. This book is based on the information I received from 116 self-identified lesbians living in Australia, who completed and returned an anonymous questionnaire during 2001 and 2002. After receiving this information I interviewed 20 lesbians from three Australian states and one Australian territory. The data collected from these women formed the basis of my PhD study, 'Lesbians' Experiences of Menopause', which I completed in 2003. This the first study to examine the topic of lesbians and menopause in Australia.

Secondly, I believe it is important that books and other information exist that speak to lesbians as well as heterosexual women. Whilst working as a nurse at a regional women's health service I was frequently asked for printed information to give to women about menopause. Sadly, the information I could find *always* assumed all women were heterosexual. In particular I searched for information that spoke to me and many of my perimenopausal lesbian friends. With the exception of one book, published in the United States, I was unable to find menopause information that did not assume heterosexuality. This is my attempt to correct this omission.

I wish to point out that this book is *not* a comparative analysis of heterosexual women's and lesbians' menopause. To write such a book would place lesbians at the margin and 'measure' them against heterosexual women, whom mainstream society deems to be the 'norm'. Many authors have written numerous academic papers, research articles and books from this dominant point of view. My book explicitly places lesbians at the centre and identifies their menopausal experiences – some of which are similar to heterosexual women's – as well as those that are unique to lesbians, as defined by lesbians themselves. My hope is that by centring lesbians' positive experiences of menopause in this way, heterosexual women may see that societal patriarchal construction (in terms of the body, notions of femininity and the negative views so often internalised about the end of our fertile years) is in fact avoidable.

Much of the existing information for midlife women focuses on the negative issues commonly associated with menopause, such as dry vaginas, painful sexual intercourse, mood swings and low libido. For many of the lesbians in my study, these issues are of little relevance and are not major concerns or problems. They assume – as I do – that menopause, like any other life stage, is a natural process. Several of the lesbians in my study commented that menopause is a time of life to be greeted with optimism and enthusiasm. It is not my intention to downplay or trivialise the difficulties some women experience at this stage of life. I acknowledge that menopause is an individual experience and for some it brings a range of physical and emotional challenges. There are many books, pamphlets, research studies, clinical trials and medical services which assist women experiencing these difficulties. This book is not a guide to menopause, nor is it a self-help manual. Rather, I discuss menopause as a social construction and focus on issues identified as important by 116 perimenopausal and postmenopausal lesbians. It is my hope that you will find something in it that speaks to you.

Acknowledgements

I was determined not to write a doctoral thesis that, apart from my supervisor, examiners and one or two friends, no one else would ever read. So I was delighted when Spinifex Press asked me if I would be interested in rewriting the thesis into a book. Having never written a book before I had little idea as to what was involved. After all, I had just written an eighty-thousand-word thesis on the same topic, so how difficult could it be? I allowed myself two months to complete the task. Now, twelve months later, the book is written and there are many women I wish to acknowledge.

To the 116 lesbians from all over Australia who trusted me with their information and stories, I owe an enormous debt. Without their participation there would not be a PhD or a book. When I felt like giving up the thesis and wondered why I was putting myself through all the stress, I reminded myself that total strangers had given their precious time to complete a questionnaire and let me interview them in the hope that something positive would happen as a result. I was determined not to waste their time. I trust that they will accept this book as my thanks and appreciation for their valuable and important contributions.

My friends and family deserve a special 'Thank you' for their love and unwavering support. For the past five years, many of our conversations have focused around lesbians and menopause. They have always been there for me, willing to discuss, debate and challenge my thoughts and ideas. In particular, I thank Monica Hingston and Peg Moran for their friendship and encouragement. My parents, Judy and John, taught me to have the courage of my convictions and to follow my dreams. My parents' love and support enriches my life. My sister Frances and I share a healthy sibling rivalry and in true rivalry fashion, she delivered a beautiful healthy baby boy (Liam James) two days after my thesis was examined. I thank her for the gift of my nephew and for asking me hard questions that cause me to re-examine and reflect on my views and attitudes.

I especially thank Renate Klein who encouraged me to begin this journey in the early 1990s. As a mature-aged, off-campus, postgraduate student struggling with the demands of work, study and life in general, Renate provided me with the support and encouragement that enabled me to continue and success-fully complete my Masters degree and later a PhD. Her belief in my ability and her passion for my topic remain a source of inspiration and motivation.

Kerry Biram has done a meticulous editing job and I thank her for her thorough work. Any errors that have slipped through remain my responsibility. I extend my sincere thanks to my publisher, Susan Hawthorne, who has been extremely supportive and encouraging throughout this entire process.

Finally, I wish to thank my partner Lesley Higgs for her patience, love and support. I am extremely fortunate to share my life with her. I look forward to many long walks on the beach with her now that the book is published.

Jennifer Kelly, Jan Juc
20 December 2004

1

Introduction

At the beginning of the twenty-first century, menopause is a frequent and hotly debated issue both in society at large and among health professionals. Nevertheless, despite the public prominence that menopause receives, the unquestioned assumption in discussions about this stage in a woman's life is that midlife women are *all* heterosexual.

The interest in this topic stems from my own experiences as both a middle-aged lesbian feminist and a long-standing women's health advocate in my work as a nurse and midwife. Starting with an issue or problem that concerns us personally is a common experience for many feminist researchers. For years I have been concerned about the ways in which many health professionals assume that all their clients, and in particular those who are older women, are heterosexual. The heterosexist[1] and indeed homophobic[2] nature of the information they present to women on the topic of menopause has long concerned and frustrated me. In this book I examine these issues as they relate to midlife lesbians.

My aim is to provide an understanding of lesbians' experiences of menopause in relation to their general health and wellbeing. By making lesbians' experiences visible through exploring the issues that are important and unique to them at this time of their lives, I hope to contribute to challenging heterosexism and homophobia within the health system and mainstream society.

This book began as my doctoral study. As this was the first Australian study into lesbians' experiences of menopause, I was keen to involve a broad group of lesbians from all over Australia. I recruited self-identified lesbians aged 39 to 65 years to my study through a variety of sources, including lesbian networks, lesbian dances and festivals, as well as the lesbian and gay media. I also recruited participants through women's health services as well as nursing journals and women's health networks, email lists and word of mouth. The most successful recruitment strategy was by word of mouth. Two hundred questionnaires were posted upon request to women throughout Australia between November 2001 and May 2002. Potential participants were sent the questionnaire accompanied by a plain language statement that explained the aims and objectives of the study. At this stage of the process I asked interested women to sign a coded consent form and I informed them that their personal details would remain confidential.

I decided to use a questionnaire as I believe it is an excellent starting point to gather statistical and other general information. Follow-up interviews were later to provide further clarification and discussion of issues identified. One hundred and twenty-four questionnaires were returned (62 per cent response rate). Eight women identified as other than lesbian (gay, homosexual, bisexual) and as a result I did not include their data in the final analysis.[3] The questionnaire was divided into six distinct parts: socio-demographic details, reproductive and menopausal health, body image, hormone replacement therapy, sex and sexuality, and health services and homophobia. I chose the first four themes, as these themes were frequently discussed in the existing literature on menopause. Feminist researchers acknowledge that women's experiences are inextricably linked to the wider socio-political environment in which we live, and for this reason I felt it was essential to include an additional theme focussing specifically on health services and homophobia. The data I collected from this section will, I believe, help in confronting and challenging homophobia within the health system.

I followed up the questionnaire data with 20 in-depth interviews. In selecting 20 lesbians to interview, I focused mainly, although not entirely, on women who identified issues for lesbians that differed from the mainstream literature. The interviews enabled me to explore and clarify many of the issues raised by the participants in the questionnaire. Out of the 124 participants who returned completed questionnaires, 110 (89 per cent) indicated their willingness to be interviewed.[4]

Participants in my study were fairly homogenous. Lesbians are, of course, as diverse as women generally, however, my sample did not reflect such diversity. Seventy-six per cent of participants were tertiary educated and almost 40 per cent of participants were employed in health-related occupations. These occupations include medical receptionists, social workers, welfare workers, personal carers, nurses, midwives, doctors, physiotherapists, occupational therapists, counsellors and other allied health professionals. As many participants are well educated and employed in the field, it might be suggested that their level of knowledge and attitudes may differ from lesbians without tertiary education and those employed in other areas.

The lesbians who returned completed questionnaires from every state and territory in Australia are not fully representative of lesbians living in Australia. The lack of a clearly defined definition of lesbian prohibits a sample from being fully representative. Gaining a truly representative sample remains a constant challenge for researchers studying groups that are marginalised and stigmatised. More studies need to be conducted with a larger sample size and with lesbians from differing races, ethnicities and socio-economic levels. The high number of lesbians working as 'insiders' in health-related occupations adds a further dimension to the study and I believe lends extra weight to these findings.

Participants' profiles

Lesbians who filled out and returned the questionnaires ranged in age from 39 to 64 years. The mean age was 49.7 years. Interviewees were aged from 46 to 60 years. The mean age of the lesbians interviewed was 51.9 years. Fifty-eight women (50 per cent of total participants) in my study were 50 years of age and over. Less than fifty-seven per cent of participants described themselves as peri-menopausal (n=66), 38.8 per cent as post-menopausal (n=45), and 4.3 per cent indicated they were unsure (n=5).

The mean number of years the women in this study identified as lesbian was 20.7. Only 17 women out of 116 had been lesbian for less than ten years. In response to the question, 'How many years have you identified as lesbian?', four women did not answer and six women wrote 'All my life'. One woman noted 'Forever'. Almost three-quarters (71 per cent) of lesbians in this study were in lesbian relationships at the time of completing the questionnaire (n=82). The length of the time women had been in their present relationship ranged between two months and 30 years. Just under half of the lesbians with partners (n=38) stated that their partner was also experiencing menopausal-related changes. This phenomenon is unique to lesbians' experiences of menopause. Table 1.1 presents a breakdown of the participants' ethnic backgrounds.

Table 1.1
PARTICIPANTS BY ETHNIC BACKGROUND

Ethnic background	Number (n)	% of sample
Australian	52	44.8
English	36	31.0
German	5	4.3
Irish	4	3.4
Welsh	2	1.7
New Zealand	2	1.7
Scottish	2	1.7
Celtic	2	1.7
Other	9	7.7
Unanswered	2	1.7
TOTAL	116	100.0

The majority of participants identified as being from Anglo-Celtic backgrounds and were living in every Australian state and territory. It is of note that there were no women of Asian background in this study.

Less than half (45 per cent) of the participants were living in the state of Victoria at the time of completing the questionnaire (n=52). The remainder of participants resided in all states and territories of Australia. Whilst the percentages of lesbians from the Australian Capital Territory and Tasmania were small, it was pleasing that the sample included lesbians from every Australian state and territory thus ensuring the study is national, rather than solely Victorian. Lesbians in this study were living in rural areas as well as capital cities. Of the 20 lesbians interviewed, 13 reside in cities and seven in rural communities. Interviewees live in Victoria (n=14), New South Wales (n=4), Australian Capital Territory (n=1) and Western Australia (n=1).

Table 1.2
PARTICIPANTS' EDUCATIONAL STATUS

Education level	n	%
Tertiary	88	75.8
Years 10–12	22	19.0
Year 9 and below	6	5.2
TOTAL	116	100.0

More than three-quarters of the participants in my study have tertiary education (n=88). Seventy-six per cent of the participants were in paid employment (n=88). Of these, 60 per cent were employed full-time, 28.4 per cent part-time and 11.3 per cent employed on a casual basis. Women were asked to rate their income level as low, medium or high. Less than 9 per cent of participants nominated high (n=10), 56 per cent indicated medium (n=65) and 35.3 per cent low (n=41).

With regard to reproductive health, 47.4 per cent of participants have given birth to their own biological children (n=55),[5] whilst 52.5 per cent do not have children (n=61). Seventeen per cent of participants have their children living with them at home (n=19) and 14 per cent of participants co-parent a child and/or children (n=16).

Eighty-six per cent of participants had a natural menopause (n=100) and 13.8 per cent had a surgical menopause (n=16). From the questionnaire responses, six of these women had their ovaries conserved, seven women had oophorectomies (ovaries removed) at the time of hysterectomy and three women did not respond to this question.

An overwhelming 87 per cent of participants in this study self-identify as feminists (n=101). Three women did not respond to this question. More than half (58 per cent) of the lesbians in this study believe there are different issues for lesbians at menopause than for heterosexual women (n=67). These specific issues will be discussed in detail in Chapter 6.

The social context of women's lives

Throughout this book, I acknowledge that women's experiences of menopause do not occur in a vacuum. Every facet of a woman's life is multifactorial and influenced by the socio-political and cultural contexts in which she lives, and menopause is no exception. My study is the first research project to focus on the menopausal experiences of lesbians living in Australia. This book draws on the experiences of 116 midlife lesbians living in Australia, who voluntarily contributed to my doctoral study.[6] Without their contributions, this book could not have been written.

Interestingly, in spite of the clear invisibility of lesbians in the menopause literature, during the course of my study I was frequently asked why I focused on lesbians' experiences of menopause. This question was then followed up with the statement that since lesbians are women, surely, lesbians' experiences of menopause would be the same as those of heterosexual women. I usually responded by saying that while this assertion may be true in terms of physiological functions, my study looks beyond the biological and physiological aspects of menopause and investigates this transition in lesbians' lives within a wider socio-political context. Nevertheless, even after explaining this rationale, some people – academic colleagues included – still persisted in asking why I would anticipate any differences between the experiences of heterosexual women and lesbians. I argue that such views highlight a profound lack of understanding of the social construction of women's different sexualities and how they influence most aspects of women's lives. I believe that these views clearly showed the necessity for this research project, as well as many more future studies on different aspects of lesbians' lives. Indeed, I claim they reflect the precise essence of the dominant, heterosexual cultural beliefs which invisibilise and discriminate against anybody who does not fit this norm (see Hawthorne, 2002).

Social contexts provide a structure for understanding our complex lives and, as such, it is important that these contexts be acknowledged and understood. In doing so, it is necessary to realise that homosexuality was only declassified as a mental illness in 1973. Prior to 1973 lesbians and gay men were looked upon as sick and deviant and, as a result, were subjected to a range of humiliating and harmful interventions in an attempt to 'treat' and 'cure' their homosexuality (Wilton, 1995). Fortunately, today homosexuality is no longer officially regarded as a mental illness; however, lesbians and gay men still experience discrimination and prejudice as a result of this earlier biological determinist model of homosexuality. As Tamsin Wilton explains, '. . . it is difficult to have faith or trust in anyone whose treatment of you is informed by her/his continued belief that your closest intimate relationships are sick, dysfunctional or abnormal' (Wilton, cited in Doyal, 1998, 153). Clearly, heterosexual women do not inhabit the same social context and therefore it may be reasonably surmised that the menopausal experiences of lesbians and heterosexual women will indeed be different.

I wish to reiterate that this book is not a comparative analysis of the experiences of menopause of heterosexual women and lesbians. In writing a book that places lesbians at the centre and focusing on the issues as determined by lesbians, I realise I am deviating from normative writing convention and for this I make no apology. Lesbians in my book are indeed located at the centre. I also realise that neither heterosexual women nor lesbians are a homogenous group and, as a result, I make no absolute claims for generalisation and/or representation.

The social construction of lesbianism

A detailed and thorough examination of the different theories of homosexuality is beyond the scope of this book,[7] however, what follows is a brief overview of the social construction of lesbianism in an attempt to contextualise my study. In doing so I follow radical feminist theory which problematises the political nature of sexuality. A fundamental premise of radical feminism is 'that women as a social group are oppressed by men as a social group and that this oppression is the primary oppression for women' (Rowland & Klein, 1996, 11). This oppression is maintained via heteropatriarchal[8] institutions and structures that include the law, medicine, family, religious institutions and marriage. Radical lesbian feminists reject the idea that heterosexuality is 'natural' and assert that it is a social and political institution, and one which restricts women's sexual self-determination and freedom (Jeffreys, 1993). For lesbian feminists, lesbianism is both a choice and an act of resistance (Jeffreys, 2003). Cheryl Clarke explains that for any woman to be a lesbian in a society that is male-supremacist, misogynist, capitalist, racist, homophobic and imperialist, this is indeed an act of bravery. As she puts it:

> No matter how a woman lives out her lesbianism – in the closet, in the state legislature, in the bedroom – she has rebelled against becoming the slave master's concubine, viz. the male-dependent female, the female heterosexual. This rebellion is dangerous in patriarchy. Men at all levels of privilege, of all classes and colours have the potential to act out legalistically, moralistically, and violently when they cannot colonize women, when they cannot circumscribe our sexual, productive, repro-ductive, creative prerogatives and energies. And the lesbian . . . has succeeded in resisting the slave master's imperialism in that one sphere of her life (1981, 128).

As a radical lesbian feminist, I argue that a range of socio-cultural and political factors, rather than simply biological factors alone, shape human sexuality. This social constructionist approach vehemently rejects the idea of sexuality as a fixed, biological and natural state and instead acknowledges that the meanings applied to sexuality differ depending upon social, political and historical contexts. This view also rejects explanations of homosexuality such as 'gay' genes, latent homosexuality, and other alleged 'causes'. Lesbian feminism in the 1970s, according to UK/Australian feminist political scientist Sheila Jeffreys '. . . transformed lesbianism from a stigmatised sexual practice into an idea and a political practice that posed a challenge to male supremacy and its basic institution of heterosexuality' (1993, ix). Unfortunately, evidence of this threat to male supremacy continues to exist even today, as I will argue in this book.

The issue of defining 'lesbian' as a category deserves some attention in this Introduction. The lack of a standard accepted definition of the term 'lesbian' has often been used as a means to dismiss or refute findings from research conducted with lesbians. Definitions of 'lesbian' differ, depending upon where and how the study samples were obtained. The term 'lesbian' embraces sexual behaviour as well as identity (Carroll, 1999). One of the most widely accepted definitions of 'lesbian' is that lesbians are '. . . women whose primary emotional and sexual relationships are with other women' (Harrison, 1996, 10). Some women may embrace the term 'lesbian', while others will not identify themselves as lesbians because of the associated stigma or fear of discrimination (Martin & Knox, 2000). As I will discuss in this book, the category of 'lesbian' is, I believe, becoming further invisibilised under the guise of the category 'queer' (see Conclusion).

British lesbian feminists Celia Kitzinger and Rachel Perkins (1993) remind us that naming is a political act. These authors argue that the labels we choose to define ourselves with reflect and compose our politics. They explain that 'to call us "lesbians" is to make one kind of political statement; to call us "gay women" or "female homosexuals" is to make a different kind of statement' (1993, 35). In an attempt to avoid the dilemmas and controversies associated with the lack of a standardised definition of the word 'lesbian', I decided early in the research process that my study would include only women who self-identified as lesbian. I received 124 completed questionnaires from women all over Australia. I find it interesting that none of the women who responded to my research identified as 'queer'. One woman identified as 'homosexual', two identified as 'gay' and five identified as 'bisexual'. As these eight women identified as 'other' than lesbian, I did not include their data in my analysis.

The medicalisation of women's lives

For a very long time, feminists have been aware and critical of the medicalisation of women's lives. It appears that every major stage in a woman's life is now under the gaze of the medical 'experts' (Crock et al., 1999). Evidence of this medicalisation is seen in adolescence where young women are frequently prescribed the contraceptive pill. The medical rationale is to regulate their periods or enable them to engage in heterosexual sex without the risk of pregnancy. However, at the same time, these young women are exposed to sexually transmitted infections and side effects of this medication. Further, medicalisation takes place in dangerous and costly infertility treatments to 'assist' infertile heterosexual 'couples' (yet these drugs and treatments are given to only half of the couple and that is women, not men). Healthy pregnancies and childbirth are now routinely 'monitored' by high technological equipment and invasive procedures. And finally, hormone replacement is prescribed to alleviate the 'symptoms' of menopause in peri-menopausal as well as postmenopausal women.

More than a decade ago feminist writers began to criticise the medicalisation of menopause. New Zealand feminist, activist and author Sandra Coney writes that the midlife woman is now, '. . . a prime target for the new prevention-orientated general practice' (1993, 15). She asserts that the medicalisation of menopause has created a new industry which enables the general practitioner (GP)[9] to feel 'active, useful and effective'. She explains:

> Research careers are being built around her, and there are doctors and medical entrepreneurs who wish to measure her bones, her breasts, the cells on her cervix and her hormone levels. People build machines that can scan, photograph, x-ray, and magnify the most intimate parts of her body. The pharmaceutical companies have a veritable chocolate box of pills, patches, pessaries, and implants for the midlife woman. She can swallow them, have them sewn into her flesh, or even insert them into her vagina – from where the magic hormones will course through her body transforming everything they touch (1993, 15).

Similarly, women's health academic and radical feminist activist Renate Klein (1992, 24) comments that as middle-aged women are diagnosed as 'walking diseases', the medical profession sees there is only one way to avoid 'menopausal misery' and that is to take HRT. Despite these and other feminists' criticisms of the medicalisation of menopause, lesbians' concerns were rarely addressed. Sandra Coney, in *The Menopause Industry* (1993), acknowledges that the heterosexual community is more restrictive in terms of allowable behaviour than the lesbian community; however, even she does not focus in any detail on lesbians' experiences of menopause.

With the increasing medicalisation of women's lives comes pressure on women to 'take control' of their health. Nancy Worcester and Mariamne Whatley, US editors of *Women's Health: Readings in Social, Economic, and Political Issues*, point out how the focus on preventative health care is a shift away from the 'sick care model' to a more individualistic, self-care model where women are targeted as major consumers of the preventative services. Health screening is heavily promoted as the responsible course of action for women to take. Indeed women are made to feel guilty if they do not avail themselves of modern technological 'advances' which cover a wide range of tests, drugs, and medical procedures (Daly, 1991). Some of these 'advances' aimed at women at midlife and beyond include bone density assessments for the detection of osteoporosis and free 'breast screening' for the early detection of breast cancer, as well as new hormonal preparations to alleviate the distressing 'symptoms' of menopause (Crock et al., 1999). Worcester and Whatley (2000, 318) argue that the successful marketing of hormones to menopausal and post-menopausal women plays on the 'fear factor'. According to these authors, '. . . fear can become an important selling point for either true prevention or early detection tests'. They point out that fear is created not only by conjuring up debilitating diseases but also by playing on women's fear of ageing.[10]

In an ageist and heterosexist society such as ours, women's experiences of growing older are not usually pleasant. There is no evidence presently available to show if lesbians internalise these negative fears of ageing, nor do we know whether lesbians, as a social group, feel differently about the use of Hormone Replacement Therapy (HRT). But many lesbians in my study articulated views that are antithetical to the medical model. As discussed in Chapter 5, based on participants' views and experiences, menopause is regarded as simply a stage in a woman's life.

As I will elaborate in this book, lesbians are reported to be less likely than heterosexual women to utilise preventative health services. This may be connected to the fact, which many feminist writers have argued, that women in general lack power in health care institutions. This impedes women's access to health care services (Doyal, 1995). In this book, I reveal additional specific problems, such as homophobia and heterosexism, which lesbians frequently encounter when accessing health services (see Chapter 5). The negative impact this has on their health and wellbeing is also addressed in that chapter. Similarly, it is not known if lesbians are more likely to use complementary or alternative medicine in preference to the Western medical model. The literature suggests this may well be the case and my study explores this issue in some detail.

Despite a growing interest in the field of women's health research, until recently very little attention has been paid to lesbian health research. This lack of literature and research on lesbian health may result in a belief that the health needs and issues of lesbian women are the same as those of other women; as a result, this leads to further invisibility of lesbians. I hope that my book will contribute to reducing this invisibility and shed new light on lesbians' health and lesbians' lives.

Lesbians, body image and menopause

When thinking of women and body image it is important to acknowledge the socio-cultural context in which women live. It is these contexts that set the rules or provide the framework for our lives. The social context in which a lesbian lives unquestionably affects every aspect of her life and therefore needs to be considered and addressed and incorporated into analyses of the different stages of her life.[1]

Many women have, for too long, had a difficult relationship with their own bodies. This difficulty, I suggest arises from living in a world where women are regarded as objects for men's desire and entertainment. US psychologist and scholar on lesbian, gay and bisexual issues, Sari Dworkin (1989) explains how men and women undergo very different socialisation processes. Dworkin highlights how girls are taught that it is their looks and actions that are deemed to be important in our society, whereas boys are taught that it is their accomplishments that matter. Sadly, these early messages are internalised and often lead women to experience negative body image for the remainder of their lives.

A number of feminists have highlighted how women are vulnerable to the 'culture of thinness' which is so pervasive in Westernised[2] society. Naomi Wolf, in the classic feminist text

The Beauty Myth, explains how the mass media is influential in communicating the messages of thinness to women across the globe. The media is said to be the barometer that women will use as the standard against which to measure themselves (Striegel-Moore et al., 1986). Women are constantly bombarded with images of the supposed ideal body weight, shape and what is considered to be attractive. As a result a large gap exists for most women between their real and desired bodies (Ludwig & Brownell, 1999). Wolf argues that the mass media has a vested interest in retaining this 'culture of thinness' as it generates multi-billion-dollar industries from women's insecurities about their physical appearance. Other feminists share this view and blame the media in part for influencing women to become obsessed with food, weight and appearance (Faludi, 1991).

It has been suggested that it might be possible for a sub-culture to reject these negative messages and, by doing so, members of the subculture will be protected from the damaging effects of a society that pressures women to conform. Lesbians are such a subculture, however, very little is known about how satisfied or dissatisfied lesbians are with their body image, as very few studies have been conducted with samples of healthy lesbians.

In the US, Maryanne Ludwig and Kelly Brownell (1999) conducted an Internet-based study to determine how self-identification as 'masculine', 'feminine' or 'androgynous' affects body image in lesbians. One hundred and eighty-eight lesbians and bisexual women participated in the study. Women were recruited via the Internet and email; they ranged in ages from 21 to 55 years. The findings revealed significant differences in body satisfaction between women who perceived themselves as masculine, feminine or androgynous. Women who rated their appearance as 'feminine' had greater body dissatisfaction than those identifying as masculine and androgynous. The authors suggest that 'feminine' women may be more susceptible than the others in the lesbian culture to cultural pressures about appearance. In addition, they argue that masculine and androgynous women may be more capable of rejecting social pressures exerted on women to conform to society's image of what a woman should look like.

Women who had mostly lesbian and bisexual women friends, rather than those with mostly heterosexual female friends, experienced the highest levels of body satisfaction. The authors claim this is due to the fact that women with mostly heterosexual friends are socialising in a group whose principles closely reflect mainstream[3] values, whereas the lesbians and bisexual women are more likely to reject and challenge the culturally prescribed notions of 'thinness' for women. This finding supports those from my own study where many lesbians claimed that a lesbian identity allowed them a sense of freedom. For example:

> Being a lesbian seems to free most women from many of the pressures that want women to conform to stereotypes of shape, beauty, fashion, etc. [67][4]

According to Sheila Jeffreys, the rejection of femininity is an important political strategy (1993). Jeffreys explains that the more women (lesbians and heterosexual) reject femininity, the easier it becomes for other women to escape these constricting and degrading feminine norms. This, she suggests, makes it more difficult to discriminate against lesbians. From many of the responses I received, it appears that several of the lesbians in my study support Jeffreys' analysis.

In a review of the literature on women and body image,[5] I found that participants in research studies exploring women and body image are frequently drawn from student populations and therefore restricted to young, white – and assumed to be heterosexual – women (see Stevens & Tiggemann, 1998). It is difficult to find information on body image in ageing women generally and, in particular, women at midlife. When researchers have looked at the issues of body image for midlife women, they have, with very few exceptions, included only the experiences of heterosexual women (Banister, 1999).

During my study, I was amazed to discover that a myth exists that lesbians are young women; it is as if, like a childhood disease, lesbianism is something we grow out of. A well-known Australian academic told me in response to my asking her how many lesbians were in her large study: 'It's [lesbianism] more common in younger women.' The audience was made up of a large number of doctors and nurses and, to my horror, no one challenged the speaker on this point. I quickly glanced around the room looking for shocked faces, however, did not see any. One woman in the audience spoke to me privately during a tea break and thanked me for asking the question. She, like me, was appalled at such a comment but felt it was not safe to challenge the 'expert' on her ignorant view.

Of the research that has looked at the issues of body image and women at midlife, the majority focuses on issues of body fat composition (Deeks, 1999). Reviewing the literature on weight changes during the menopausal years reveals many inconsistencies and often leaves the reader bewildered. Some studies report that weight gain at the time of menopause is not directly related to menopause, while others suggest that menopause may have a direct effect on weight (see Crawford et al., 2000). The issue of Hormone Replacement Therapy (HRT)[6] is often discussed in relation to weight gain at midlife, however, once again the information is often inconsistent and contradictory (see Chapter 4 for further discussion of HRT).

What the research tells us

Women are more dissatisfied with their bodies than men, so the research from many countries tells us. The dissatisfaction among women is so common that this phenomenon has even been given a name. In a study focussing on women and weight, researchers Judith Rodin, Lisa Silberstein and Ruth Striegel-

Moore coined the term 'normative discontent'. Women are now said to suffer from 'normative discontent' (Rodin et al., 1985). This, I suggest, is another example of the many ways society pathologises and medicalises almost every part of a woman's life. It is well known that a woman's physical appearance changes as a result of the ageing process, but how women feel about these age-related changes is not really understood. In my own study I was keen to learn how lesbians felt about the bodily changes they experience at the time of menopause.

Throughout the course of my study, I found that the results of many larger published studies and the findings from my sample often differed enormously. Many of the issues mentioned in the mainstream literature that were said to be of importance to women often appeared to be of little importance and/or relevance to many of the lesbians in my study.

Studies that include sexual orientation suggest that lesbians may have a better body image than their heterosexual counterparts (Gettelman & Thompson, 1993; Siever, 1994; Bergeron & Senn, 1998). Could it be true that lesbians somehow manage to escape the prescriptive models of the media, medicine and menopause? As one respondent to my questionnaire wrote:

> Women who accept themselves as they are don't have to prove anything about their appearance. Lesbians are less tied into the social pressure, i.e. thin bodies. [34]

Although such studies are scarce, some researchers have suggested that a lesbian identity may protect lesbians from the devastating effects of a society which pressures women to be thin (Bergeron & Senn, 1998). Results from my study neither totally confirm nor reject this notion. Sherry Bergeron and Charlene Senn compared the attitudes of lesbians and heterosexual women towards their bodies and investigated the relationship between body dissatisfaction and the ways in which women took on board these negative messages. In this Canadian study, 108 lesbians and 116 heterosexual women aged between 18 and 58 years completed and returned a questionnaire. The results support previous research, which states that lesbians are generally less dissatisfied with their bodies than are their heterosexual counterparts. The authors found that heterosexual women had a thinner ideal body than the lesbians. Lesbians felt stronger and fitter than the heterosexual women in the study. Lesbians were less concerned with the size of their thighs and buttocks than the heterosexual women, which the researchers claim is '. . . the result of lesbians' resistance to social norms about this part of their bodies' (1998, 397). The authors conclude by stating that there is support for the idea that a lesbian identity, although it does not 'immunise' lesbians against the devastating effects of the 'culture of thinness', does, however, act as a 'buffer' which limits the internalisation of these societal norms.

I asked women in my study if they believed a lesbian identity protected them from the desire to be thin. Responses to this question were varied. Over a quarter of the participants agreed that a lesbian identity might protect lesbians from the desire to be thin, while 46 per cent disagreed with this suggestion. Another 26 per cent were unsure, and two participants did not respond to this question. Women's responses to my questionnaire data which support the view that a lesbian identity may protect lesbians from the desire to be thin, include:

> I don't desire to be thin – just comfortable and healthy with my body. I stopped worrying about thin/fat as an image long ago. This is partly due to a feminist view and lesbian influences. [25]

Similarly, another woman wrote:

> I still like my body regardless of the sagging breasts, varicose veins and age spots on the back of my hands. Some lesbians I know are very weight conscious, diet, display anxiety about their weight and openly criticise others they consider fat. I

believe they have been socialised into accepting that thin is beautiful in the same way that heterosexual women have. [1]

Quite obviously lesbians, like heterosexual women, are exposed to society's negative messages. However, some lesbians seem to protect themselves from these views in some specific areas. It was clear from several of the responses in my study that many lesbians were resisting body shape pressure because of a political stance. An overwhelming 87 per cent of lesbians (101) in my study self-identify as feminists and therefore it is not surprising that the majority of their responses reflect a feminist analysis. Feminists have for a long time been aware that fat is, indeed, a feminist issue (Orbach, 1978).

Despite these positive comments which indicate a healthy approach towards body image, other responses reflect a common dissatisfaction with one's body. Lesbians, too, are vulnerable to the 'culture of thinness'.

I don't like fat arms, no waist, cellulite on my legs. I have drawn and painted women's bodies all of my life and I enjoy the sexiness of youth. I resent that this [menopause] has happened about 10 years before it should have. At 50 I could cope but in my early 40s I feel cheated and unable to start again. [125]

I am afraid of looking old and [having] grey hair and I do not want to be an old bitter person and all alone. I think young and try hard to hang on to my youth. I need it now. My son keeps me young inside. [157]

For some, it is a challenge to balance different life demands:

I am not entirely satisfied. I feel that my weight gain is a sign that I have let myself go. At a time in my life when I have the time and finances to indulge in fine food, the universe has conspired to slow my metabolic rate and not allow me to indulge as frequently as I would like. [198]

It is interesting to note that many of the lesbians who have a negative body image indicated that they had been in previous long-term heterosexual relationships. As I did not specifically ask all of the study participants whether they had been in previous long-term heterosexual relationships, I cannot make any representational claims. However, while this is a small sample and not representative of the population of lesbians generally, perhaps some of the lesbians who had been previously married and led 'conventional' heterosexual lives may be more likely to be affected by the negative effects of a patriarchal society which pressures women to conform, in other words, to be thin. It became clear to me from the self-disclosure of issues in their previous married lives that some women's responses and attitudes towards their bodies appear to be framed through a heterosexual lens.

I was astounded and found it quite disturbing that during the interviews some of the lesbians displayed extremely homophobic attitudes and reinforced many of mainstream society's negative views of lesbians. These views are somewhat understandable, as I'm sure any lesbian or gay man knows that it is virtually impossible not to take on at least some of society's negative messages about our sexual orientation. Celia Kitzinger in *The Social Construction of Lesbianism* (1987) explains how studies about members of stigmatised and oppressed groups consistently reveal accounts in which these members accept the majority stereotype. This internalisation of negative attitudes about our lesbian or gay orientation has been termed 'internalized homophobia' (Malyon, 1982).

British researchers Celia Kitzinger and Rachel Perkins are highly critical of this terminology as they argue it pathologises lesbian oppression. 'Therapists tell us that as a direct consequence of our oppression in an anti-lesbian world, we are sick and in need of cure' (1993, 101). These authors assert that when lesbians refuse to be defined and controlled by men, lesbians are a real threat to heteropatriarchy and consequently '. . . we experience hatred, fear, aggression, derision, rejection, marginalisation, as a direct consequence of being lesbian. Is it any wonder that at times we don't like being lesbian very much?' (1993, 103). Kitzinger and Perkins believe that the result of using this terminology is to depoliticise lesbians' oppression and, instead, reduce it to an individual psychological problem, which requires individual rather than social change (1993, 104). While I do not wish to depoliticise lesbians' oppression and blame the individual lesbian for her internalised negative views, it is obvious that some of the lesbians in my study unfortunately hold extremely negative and homophobic views. In a follow-up interview to filling in the questionnaire, Janet[7] asserted:

Some lesbians go out of their way to make themselves unattractive and they hide behind a victim façade. A lot of women aren't completely OK within themselves or have low self-esteem. They kind of band together in a tribal sort of group; while I'm not criticising them, it's just not how I work myself. Some lesbians like to look alike which I don't actually find attractive myself. To me they just don't seem to want to make themselves look attractive. People should make an effort to look their best. I think it is a sign of self-esteem and self-awareness. [170]

Although disturbing and reflective of the view that being 'attractive' meant attractiveness as defined within the dominant hetero-patriarchal culture, the majority of lesbians in my study did not share this view. Nevertheless, Jess relayed similar ideas:

. . . some lesbians are under pressure not to look straight, e.g., you are not a 'real' lesbian if you wear makeup or carry a handbag. I don't go around looking like a tizzy straight person. I never wear a dress but I don't believe in a uniform for anybody. You can still run around looking like Margaret Thatcher; she's someone who just popped into mind, because she used to wear pearls. It is easier for identification purposes if you have a dress code rather than trying to suss people out all of the time. But I don't believe in putting people under pressure to all have short haircuts, carry a wallet in your back pocket, but if you want to be like that . . . it's just not me. [180]

As noted earlier, an interesting observation is that both these women disclosed that they had previously been in long-term heterosexual marriages. As this issue was beyond the scope of this study, these matters were not investigated in any further detail. The majority of responses, however, did not reflect such negative attitudes. Many of the lesbians interviewed held opposing viewpoints and drew a strong connection between their feminist identity and healthy body image. Despite the high percentage of feminists in my sample, their attitudes towards their bodies were not, in all cases, always positive. These findings support those of other studies, which did not confirm the notion that a feminist ideology necessarily leads to a more positive body image. From many of the participants' responses, however, it appears that a feminist identity certainly does provide some protection from these patriarchal standards of femininity. That the body is important to lesbians can be seen in a whole range of artistic works produced by lesbians, many of which either challenge normative models of the feminine body or present the lesbian in intimate and loving ways.

Several of the lesbians I interviewed spoke of the importance of physical attractiveness for women in sexual relationships with men. US feminist researcher Esther Rothblum explains how, for women who do not relate sexually to men, physical attractiveness is not such an issue (Rothblum, 1994). In my study, in response to a question that asked if there are any differences for lesbians at menopause compared with the experiences of heterosexual women, Sulo wrote that there is less pressure to maintain that youthful look. In an interview she elaborated:

This is very subjective but it seems to me – and I don't want to idealise it – that lesbians are more interested in the sort of friendship and spiritual quality of the relationship than in a heterosexual relationship where your looks and sex appeal is more important to men than it is to women. That is my own feeling towards my partner. I want to maintain my health and fitness and it may be because of that we are concerned about how much weight we are gaining rather than just about the way we look. [26]

Similarly, Anne wrote that 'a strong feminist look is more important than physical attractiveness'. Anne explains:

A youthful look is just that but an old woman has the road maps of where she's been as well as in her whole being, in particular on her face as well. I think we, as lesbians, don't have this stereotype that the blonde bimbo is the person that is necessarily the one we find attractive. So an older woman, because of who she is rather than having a Barbie doll figure, is what we are more likely to be attracted to, and the whole person. It's not just the physical part; it's the attractiveness of the whole personality too. I think this isn't the case for men picking partners. They still have to be leering over another person, and porn stuff. I think we have the capacity to get beyond that. So as an older person, I don't think you feel as though you are on the shelf as such because it's from that point of view. [81]

Joy continued this theme and spoke of the ways many heterosexual women consider themselves less sexual, less useful and less attractive to men at menopause. During the interview with me, Joy expanded on this theme:

My heterosexual friends who are getting to menopause are quite unhappy about it because it signifies the end of something for them. I don't know whether them being childbearing makes them more attractive to men. I don't know exactly about that because I haven't done it. These are very close friends, women

25

I have known all my life. Well, they talk now like it is normal. I mean, when I told them I was in menopause they did a 'feeling sorry for me' lot of sounds rather than, 'oh great'. And I said, 'Oh no, this is really good'. But for them it is a sign of ageing. Being older as a heterosexual isn't very attractive, if you are a woman. For them, they are apparently not sought after. The heterosexual culture goes for the young look, as we all know. And in lesbian culture, I haven't found that. Quite a few of us are looking forward to not bleeding; quite a few of us are making jokes about 'royal flushes' and things like that. Two of my heterosexual friends were quite negative about it without actually articulating why they were negative. It was almost as if it were a normalised internal negativity. [68]

I asked participants in my study about the level of satisfaction with their present body shape, size and weight. Interestingly, fitness appeared to be much more important than physical attractiveness, as is illustrated in the following quotations:

I am more concerned about my physical fitness than attractiveness as I believe one leads to the other. [199]

I don't crave the perfect body – never have. I carry a few extra kilos but I am physically fit and I don't see this as a problem. I like my body and what it does. I enjoy an active life and fitness is important. [101]

I have always set out to maintain a fairly physically fit body. I see physical fitness as a strength. [8]

I don't think 'thin' is important, but I think 'fit' is. I need to shape up for the Gay Games in 2002. [134]

This focus on fitness and strength was a common recurring theme throughout both the questionnaires and interview responses yet it is rarely mentioned in the mainstream literature on women and body image. There is also much research on the health-promoting effects of strength training and many older women are now actively participating in strength training programs. Miriam Nelson in her book *Strong Women, Strong Bones* (2000) discusses the benefits of such programs regarding bone health and the prevention of osteoporosis. Other reported benefits of strength training include improved muscle strength, balance and coordination. Regular physical activity is also associated with improved psychosocial health, as it is understood that physical activity reduces anxiety, depression and improves mood (US Department of Health and Human Services, 1996). A recent study in Victoria, Australia, showed that only 51 per cent of women were sufficiently active to promote health and guard against disease. This study also showed that the levels of physical inactivity increase along with women's age (Smith et al., 1999). If fitness is regarded as a higher priority for lesbians than for heterosexual women, therefore lesbians are more physically active, it could be suggested that lesbians might enjoy a physically healthier old age. It is vital that these health-promoting messages are spread widely across the general community so that all women may benefit from this knowledge.

It is important for us to question the type of research that is conducted, as not all research is 'good' research. Much of the existing research on lesbians and body image is in relation to lesbians with eating disorders. Research comparing heterosexual women with lesbians has revealed differences and often comes up with conflicting results. US feminist psychologist Laura S Brown (1987) contends that lesbians appear less likely to have eating disorders than women generally. The literature, however, is scarce and it is clear that more studies need to be conducted with healthy, non-clinical samples of lesbians at midlife and across the lifespan to find out more.

When compared with heterosexual women, Thomas Gettelman and J Kevin Thompson (1993) found that lesbians were less concerned with weight, dieting and issues of body image. The researchers looked at differences among homosexual and heterosexual males and females on issues of body image disturbance and concerns about weight gain and eating disturbances. The study sample was made up of 32 homosexual males, 32 homosexual females, 32 heterosexual males and 32 heterosexual females.

Findings indicated that heterosexual females, along with homosexual males, displayed greater anxiety with appearance, weight, dieting and had greater body image disturbances compared to heterosexual males and homosexual females. Lesbians in this study reported fewer body image problems than heterosexual females and homosexual males. These findings are consistent with those of other published studies (Cash & Brown, 1989; Herzog, et al., 1992; Rothblum, 1994; Siever, 1994) and indeed support the findings from my own study.

It seems obvious that the common feature shared by heterosexual females and homosexual males is their desire to attract and please men. Clearly lesbians (and heterosexual men) are not looking for men's attention or approval, and therefore they are not concerned about these issues that are defined and prescribed by men under patriarchy. Given this analysis, it is hardly surprising to learn that in this study, heterosexual women displayed the greatest anxiety about being overweight.

Gettelman and Thompson also found that dieting was more common among the heterosexual women. Heterosexual women also displayed the highest level of eating disturbances compared with all other groups. The authors state that as previous research comparing heterosexual and homosexual females on measures of body image and disturbance is inconsistent, it is not possible to draw any definite conclusions as to why lesbians have fewer problems about body image and dieting. They suggest that a possible explanation is that lesbians may be trying to achieve different physical standards from those of heterosexual women. The authors propose that in establishing a lesbian identity, lesbians might resist the narrow and restrictive heterosexually prescribed mould for themselves, which many believe to be indicative of male oppression (1993, 551). Rather than adhering to these culturally determined 'norms', lesbians may embrace a wider range of sizes, shapes and appearances. I believe that these results were supported by many of the lesbians in my study as they were consciously rejecting the culturally determined norms and embracing a much healthier and diversified range of sizes, shapes and appearances. Quotations from my questionnaire and interview data have illustrated how, for many lesbians, the culturally determined norms are irrelevant and of little if any importance to them.

Looking at other research conducted on this topic, a Canadian study by Elizabeth Banister (1999) examined the meaning of midlife experiences in relation to women's own interpretations of their changing bodies. Acknowledging the misconceptions that exist around women's midlife period and the effects of ageism and sexism, Banister interviewed eleven women aged 40–53 years, exploring the physiological and socio-cultural factors underlying their experiences.

Although this was a small sample, it included women who are generally under-represented in health research. In terms of racial background, nine women identified as white, one as Aboriginal, and one as Asian. Five of the participants were married, one had never married, and five were divorced or separated. Two of the participants were lesbians. Except for one woman, all participants had children.

The findings indicate that although physical health matters are important at this stage of life, it is actually the socio-cultural context in which these issues are understood that is problematic (1999, 531). Banister explains: 'This context defines the ways in which midlife women engage with their health issues' (1999, 531). Much of the existing mainstream research, I suggest, does not acknowledge the important role context plays in women's lives. Feminism is also a socio-cultural context and it undoubtedly affects how women think, act and behave in the world. Feminism influences every aspect of our lives. When feminism is added to lesbian existence, these two forces together enhance behavioural change, which increases the likelihood of resisting cultural norms and further of creating, within lesbian communities, new norms which go against the mainstream. Adrienne Rich (1980), in her famous essay 'Compulsory Heterosexuality and Lesbian Existence', explains how lesbian existence is the rejection of a way of life. She asserts:

> Lesbian existence comprises both the breaking of a taboo and the rejection of a way of life. It is also a direct or indirect attack on male right of access to women. But it is more than these, although we may first begin to perceive it as a form of nay saying to patriarchy, an act of resistance. It has of course included role playing, self hatred, breakdown, alcoholism, suicide and intra-woman violence; we romanticise at our peril what it means to love and act against the grain, and under heavy penalties; and lesbian existence has been lived (unlike say Jewish or Catholic existence) without access to any knowledge of a tradition, a continuity, a social underpinning. The destruction of records and memorabilia and letters documenting the realities of lesbian existence must be taken very seriously as a means of keeping heterosexuality compulsory for women, since what has been kept from our knowledge is joy, sensuality, courage and community, as well as guilt, self-betrayal and pain (Rich, 1981, 24).

By rejecting the narrowly defined socio-cultural norms that have been prescribed under patriarchy, lesbians are now free to create and embrace other norms. Lesbian feminism offers and provides a new vibrant way of being in the world. It gives sense, joy and purpose to many lesbians' lives.

A South Australian community study conducted by Claire Stevens and Marika Tiggemann (1998) also supported previous research findings that women in the general population are dissatisfied with their bodies and desire to be thinner. This study found that women's dissatisfaction with their bodies was constant across the ages of 18–59 years, and factors such as marital status, education level and occupational status did not affect the level of dissatisfaction. The authors acknowledge the bias inherent in their study as '. . . nearly all of the participants were Caucasian' (1998, 100). Unfortunately, sexual orientation was neither included nor discussed. Participants were not asked about their sexual orientation and the researchers noted only that 71 per cent were married, 21 were living with a partner and 31 described themselves as single (1998, 96). Marital status was viewed as an important variable in determining the emphasis placed on attractiveness, as '. . . single women are more likely than their married counterparts to try to be attractive to men' (1998, 96). Heterosexual bias is therefore obvious, however, it is not acknowledged. Sadly, this heterosexual bias appears to be the norm in research studies today.

Joan Chrisler and Laurie Ghiz (1993) assert that regardless of whether menopause is viewed as a positive or negative occurrence, it certainly changes how women perceive their bodies. In response to my question, 'Has your experience of menopause changed the way you view yourself', almost 58 per cent of participants indicated 'Yes'. Similarly, 85 per cent of participants had noticed their body shape changing. Of these, 64 per cent were concerned about these changes, while 36 per cent were not. As illustrated above, lesbians reflect both negative and positive body image issues.

While my study is not a comparative analysis between heterosexual women and lesbians, the findings do yield interesting results regarding body image, and support the findings of other researchers that lesbians may be striving to maintain different physical ideals from those of heterosexual women (Gettelman & Thompson, 1993). Although all women experience societal pressure to be thin, this effect appears more pronounced among heterosexual women than among lesbians (Brand et al., 1992). The emphasis placed on fitness, and the fact that over a quarter of the lesbians in my sample had noticed their body shape changing and yet were not concerned about these changes, tends to support this view. This is indeed good news, as it shows that many lesbians are living happy, healthy and satisfied lives at the time of menopause.

In summary, on the topic of body image, both the questionnaire and interview data from my study indicate that within this group of lesbians there exists a wide range of views and experiences relating to lesbians' satisfaction levels with their body image. Clearly, a feminist and/or lesbian identity does not provide automatic immunity to the 'culture of thinness', however, a lesbian identity may act as a buffer to the internalisation of these socio-cultural norms (Bergeron & Senn, 1998, 398). Some lesbians who disclosed that they had lived in long-term heterosexual relationships expressed views that may be regarded as homophobic and anti-lesbian. These results tend to support some of the findings from other published studies, while also adding new information and providing ideas for further research.

Lesbian identity appears to have a positive effect on a woman's image of herself. This suggests that the experience of lesbians at midlife and in old age may vary significantly from that which is regarded as the norm in mainstream society, and in medical and social research. If that is so, then the experiences of lesbians might also prove that the so-called 'norm' is no such thing, but rather a constructed view which can be challenged, and *is* challenged by the lesbians who took part in this study. I suggest that there are lessons to be learnt from the lesbians who participated in my study. Many of their responses have illustrated how resisting and rejecting patriarchal norms is indeed a health enhancing behaviour. In the next chapter, I expand upon this theme and discuss the issues related to sex and sexuality at menopause.

3

Sex and sexuality at menopause

In societies constructed by misogyny, the act of loving a woman
is revolutionary; loving ourselves as women, loving another
woman as sexual partner, loving women as a class undermines
the hegemony of male favoritism. To love woman, love
womanly, has no social support in heteropatriarchy, therefore it
must spring from some impulse within us; it must come from
itself.[1]

Sex and sexuality are important topics and it is crucial to
distinguish between the terms 'sex' and 'sexuality' as they are
often incorrectly used interchangeably. Much of the medical
literature, for example, uses the term sexuality, when in fact it
is referring to sexual activity. Throughout this book I use the
term 'sex' when speaking of sexual activity and 'sexuality' to
include all of the attitudes, beliefs, values and behaviours that
are regarded as having sexual significance in our society (see
Jackson & Scott, 1996, 2).

The vast majority of women, if they live long enough, will
experience menopause. However, when I reviewed the
literature on sex and sexuality at menopause, once again I was
struck by the lack of mention of lesbians in the research. Until
recently, very few studies have looked at menopause from the

point of view of women's personal experiences, and even fewer from a lesbian perspective. As lesbians' experiences are largely excluded from the research on sex and sexuality at midlife, little is thus known about menopause and its effects on the sexuality of lesbians. In my study I set out to start correcting this exclusion and in doing so I discovered some new, exciting and challenging insights.

Sexual disinterest or sexual dysfunction?

A review of the literature on (heterosexual) women's sexual experiences at menopause reveals a concern with issues of sexual functioning (usually referred to as 'dysfunction'), arousal time and dry vaginas. Male partners' sexual problems feature prominently in many studies of women and sex at menopause.[2] This is in stark contrast to my research, which does not focus on sexual dysfunction or partner problems. I will highlight the differences between my study and mainstream research by providing a brief overview of the mainstream literature.

In an article by Morris Gelfand, 'Sexuality among older women', he estimates the incidence of so-called sexual dysfunction in women to be between 25 and 63 per cent (2000, S20). Gelfand acknowledges that this difference is based on whether the studies are community-based or conducted with women attending menopause clinics. He cites several factors that may have a negative impact on sexual activity in menopausal women. The first he discusses is (male) partner availability. The fact that women are outliving men ('84 men for every 100 women aged between 65 and 69 years of age') according to Gelfand (2000, S19) appears to be a major contributor to negative sexual feelings experienced by women. Gelfand is assuming that the loss of a woman's husband or long-term heterosexual partner automatically results in negative sexual feelings. He does not, however, provide qualitative data to support this claim. Gelfand mentions other factors contributing to women's negative feelings around sexual activity; these include: impotence in men, alterations in libido, issues of poor general health, depression and effects of medication, dyspareunia (painful sexual intercourse) in women and decreased hormone levels. In many sexuality studies it is unquestionably implied that *all* midlife women need or even desire a male partner in order to have a healthy sex life. It is seldom considered that some women actually prefer to have sexual relationships with women. Yet again it appears there is only *one* form of sexuality, which is 'compulsory hetero-sexuality' (Rich, 1980).

Another survey found that the prevalence of alleged sexual dysfunction among women aged 18 to 59 years is 43 per cent (Laumann et al., 1999). Although this statistic is repeatedly cited in popular as well as medical literature on women's sexuality in the US, UK, Australia and other Westernised countries, its accuracy is highly questionable. This figure arose from a survey conducted in 1992 in the USA, in which 1500 women were asked questions such as whether they had ever experienced a lack of desire for sex, or anxiety related to sexual performance over the past twelve months. Women who said 'Yes' to any of these questions were characterised as suffering from Female Sexual Dysfunction (FSD). I would argue that not wanting sex once or even a few times over a whole year does not amount to a 'dysfunction'! It must also be noted that the researchers exploring FSD were funded by Pfizer, the manufacturers of Viagra (Dow, 2003).

Roy Moynihan, an Australian journalist based in the US, explained in an editorial of the *British Medical Journal* in 2003 how drug companies invented a new disease, Female Sexual Dysfunction (FSD), in an attempt to create a market for the female version of the highly lucrative drug, Viagra (sildenafil citrate). In his editorial, Moynihan details seven scientific meetings, dating back to 1997, all but one supported by a large number of pharmaceutical companies. As he puts it, 'A cohort of researchers with close ties to drug companies are working with colleagues in the pharmaceutical industry to develop and define a new category of human illness at meetings heavily sponsored by companies racing to develop new drugs' (2003, 45). He points out how specialists have been working to create a definition of a condition in order for new drugs and clinical trials to be created and designed.

Leonore Tiefer, a psychiatrist at New York University, convened a group of clinicians and social scientists in 2000 to discuss the issue of the creation of this new 'disorder', FSD, and to develop feminist responses to it. A working group was formed which co-authored a document entitled 'A New View of Women's Sexual Problems'. This document marked the beginning of an educational campaign aimed at challenging the myths of female sexual dysfunction promoted by the pharmaceutical industry (Tiefer et al., 2002).

Tiefer and her colleagues critique the accepted American Psychiatric Association definition of sexual dysfunction, which was created in 1980 for the *Diagnostic and Statistical Manual of Mental Disorders* (DSM). The working group emphasises the problematic nature of the medical model in defining women's sexual problems as it '. . . reduces sexual problems to universalized disorders of physiological function, comparable to breathing or digestive disorders' (2002, 226). They also stress the fact that women are seldom asked to discuss their sexual experiences from their own point of view and in their own words, and when they are consulted, their accounts differ vastly from men's. The authors explain how the focus on genital and physiological similarities between men and women disregards the effect of personal sexual experience and social inequalities relating to class, gender, sexual orientation and ethnicity. Women's social, political and economic situations all impact upon their ability to experience sexual health, pleasure and satisfaction, however, when using a biomedical framework to diagnose female sexual dysfunction these issues are totally ignored. Such a reductionist, biomedical model does not acknowledge relationship and intimacy as well as the accompanying power issues between men and women, which, as the working group note, are often the underlying reasons behind sexual dissatisfaction and/or displeasure.[3] Clearly, a new definition of women's sexual problems is needed. The working group defines women's sexual problems as 'discontent or dissatisfaction with any emotional, physical or relational aspect of sexual experience' (2002, 229).

Sexuality and the effects of hormones

The study of the relationship between a woman's hormonal status and her sexuality has been a popular theme for many decades. From menarche[4] through to menopause a woman is commonly seen to be at the mercy of her hormones – which are often blamed for her 'emotional' or 'irrational' behaviour. It is thus not surprising that much of the current medical research on menopause and sexuality focuses on the 'obvious' role hormones play at midlife.

Philip Sarrel (2000, S25) suggests that altered sexual function in postmenopausal women is '. . . at least in part due to hormone deficiency'. He argues that as the majority of women experience changes in their sexual function at this time when hormonal production is diminishing, there is reason to believe that hormones are partly responsible. Other external factors that may have a major effect on a woman's sexuality are rarely considered. Because of his belief in the role of hormones, his conclusion that Hormone Replacement Therapy (HRT) is capable of restoring previous levels of sexual desire and function is to be expected.

However, in another study by the same researcher, 252 naturally menopausal women were evaluated for the efficacy of HRT use on vaginal dryness, dyspareunia and decreased libido. Interestingly, the results showed that there were very few differences in the numbers of sexual complaints between the women taking HRT and those who were not. The author points out that none of the women were using androgen (testosterone) therapy (2000, S28). Sarrel then concludes that women who use androgen replacement therapy as well as HRT might experience significant higher rates of sexual desire, arousal, fantasies and frequency of sexual intercourse and orgasm than women using oestrogen alone.

Indeed, surveying the international literature, it is obvious that the effects of hormones on women's sexuality appear to be a popular focus of international biomedical research. In an Australian study conducted by Susan Davis (1998), the effects of estradiol[5] alone versus estradiol and testosterone implants in 33 postmenopausal women were compared over a two-year period. Women receiving the combined estradiol and testosterone implants reported improved sexual satisfaction, pleasure and orgasm compared with women given estradiol alone. However, as Davis cautions correctly, testosterone therapy 'is only of benefit in terms of sexuality to women who have a significant hormonal component to their sexual dysfunction' (1998, 157), thus at least acknowledging the possibility of social factors impinging on a woman's sex life. Further research is underway exploring the long-term effects of androgen on sexual desire in women, however, no questions about sexual orientation are being asked. Yet again, it appears that sexual orientation remains an unacknowledged variable.

In an earlier Australian study researchers examined the effects of oestrogen treatment and other hormones on women's sexual interest, responsiveness and frequency of sexual intercourse (Dennerstein et al., 1980). The researchers found that decreased oestrogen had a negative impact on sexual interest and activity, and oestrogen therapy had a positive impact on sexual interest and sexual response. The research team did not, however, find an increase in the frequency of intercourse as a result of oestrogen therapy and suggested further attention needed to be given to the *male* partner when assessing issues of frequency of sexual intercourse. In a more recent study, it was found that:

> . . . no relationship was evident between HRT use and any of the parameters of sexual functioning, even vaginal dryness/dyspareunia. This may well suggest that the type of HRT used may not be well adapted towards providing optimal sexual outcomes (Dennerstein et al., 1999, 260).

Once again we see how much of the mainstream (hetero-sexual) literature identifies male partner problems as one of the key determinants in women's decreased interest in sex at this stage of their lives (Gelfand, 2000; Hawton, 1994; Sarrel, 1982). The results from my own study highlighted many different findings, not surprisingly, given that the study centred on lesbians' experiences of menopause. Indeed the information gained from the questionnaire and interview responses in my study sheds new light on the heterosexist and medicalised approach to sex and sexuality at the time of menopause. These views will follow later in this chapter (see pp. 48–63), however, the following quote from one of my study participants puts the research discussed into perspective:

> . . . it is difficult when talking about lesbian sex to define it only as vaginal sex similar to hetero-sex. My intimacy is just as intense and important to me in my relating. [72]

From my extensive searching, I discovered there is very little research conducted which acknowledges lesbians as a separate group of women within the research samples. In late 2002, the Jean Hailes Foundation[6] was recruiting participants for a large study to evaluate the responses of women to a sexual satisfaction questionnaire and determine whether this questionnaire could differentiate women who are sexually satisfied from women who are sexually dissatisfied. The Subject Information Sheet reads:

Women who are sexually active (in some form) on average once a fortnight may participate in this study. We will not inquire as to the specific nature of your sexual activity. What is important for us to determine is whether or not the experience is pleasurable and satisfying. We also will not inquire about the gender of your partner or the quality of your relationship as our primary focus is to develop a measure of the isolated sexual experience. We aim to recruit 200 premenopausal and 200 postmenopausal women.

The study's research coordinator explained to me that by not asking for information regarding partners' gender or quality of relationship, the study is respecting the women's privacy and the study outcome will not be affected (personal communication, 2002). She did not regard this deliberate omission as an example of heterosexism or homophobia. Similarly, she did not regard the inclusion of qualitative information such as the woman's feelings towards her partner (if indeed there even is a partner!) or the social context in which the woman lives, as necessary variables in their study. I would argue that the failure to acknowledge the socio-cultural context in which the woman lives is likely to provide inaccurate and misleading research findings. I discussed this issue with her, however, she did not see any problem associated with the study design and dismissed my concerns.

This would have been, in my view, an ideal opportunity to acknowledge and include lesbians as a separate group of women, in an attempt to learn if the issues experienced by heterosexual women also apply to lesbians. My study, as well as large amounts of anecdotal evidence, leads me to suggest that heterosexual women experience levels of sexual dissatisfaction at much higher rates than lesbians. However, without any published studies and data to support my suggestion, once again lesbians' experiences remain invisible. This knowledge is important because if it is found that lesbians have higher sexual satisfaction levels, and less anxiety related to menopause and sexual issues, then this information needs to be widely known. I believe that women deserve to know that there are alternatives to what mainstream society would have us believe is our destiny. Lesbianism is such an alternative.

While researchers frequently justify the omission of sexual orientation as 'respecting the woman's privacy', I believe this omission is in fact due to a fear of offending and alienating heterosexual women. (See Chapter 5 for further discussion of offending heterosexual women.) In all of the studies discussed above, heterosexuality is taken for granted. When sexuality is mentioned and investigated, it is *always* heterosexuality.

Decreasing oestrogen levels seem to be a cause of loss of vaginal lubrication in some women at midlife. Surprisingly, given this information, Myra Hunter (1990) reported that less than half of postmenopausal women experienced vaginal dryness as a problem during intercourse and only a quarter of premenopausal and perimenopausal women noted this as a concern. Another determinant of vaginal lubrication as noted by Linda Gannon (1999) is the frequency and regularity of sexual activity. Rosetta Reitz (1977) claims that women who masturbate regularly, as compared to those who masturbate occasionally, report increased vaginal lubrication with a partner and decreased pain due to dryness. It has been suggested that too often various forms of HRT are considered as the first line of 'treatment' for vaginal dryness when other non-hormonal preparations also prove effective (Gannon, 1999). Other feminist researchers are aware of these 'alternatives' yet unfortunately these 'alternative' options are rarely promoted.

Shere Hite, long-time US feminist and researcher on female sexuality, argues that women do not need drugs in order to be sexually aroused. Hite suggests that a new approach to human intimacy is needed, one in which understandings of sexual expression extend beyond the limits of sexual intercourse. Hite's research identifies a lack of orgasm during sex as the most common reason for women's dissatisfaction and disenchantment in sex. To this end, she asks that more attention be paid to masturbation, rather than medication. As she puts it:

> . . . the overwhelming majority of women, according to my research, can have orgasms easily during masturbation so why not during coitus? The answer is that during masturbation women chose to stimulate the clitoral or pubic area. Only rarely – in 2 per cent of cases – does it involve vaginal penetration. In other words, the stimulation women give themselves to reach orgasm is – unlike that used by men – radically different from the stimulation most women receive during coitus (Hite, 2003, 11).

It appears obvious from Hite's research that another form of sexual expression is needed and indeed warranted. Hite concludes her article with the following comments:

> Women know how to have orgasms but do not feel free to express this during sex with men. It's not arousal pills we need, but a whole new kind of physical relations with each other (2003, 11).

Clearly lesbian sexuality is a satisfying, valid and meaningful form of sexual expression. For reasons I will discuss in the following section, this option is never encouraged or even suggested in many popular or scientific articles. Fortunately, however, many women are aware of lesbianism as a valid form of sexual expression and way of life. Findings from my study illustrate that for many lesbians, the sexual problems and difficulties highlighted in research studies and published in academic journals with heterosexual women are irrelevant. So why are lesbians' views not known more widely?

Nett Hart, in her essay 'From an eroticism of difference to an intimacy of equals: A radical feminist lesbian separatist perspective on sexuality' (Hart, 1996, 69) explains how women loving women threatens and weakens the hegemony of male bias. Consequently, lesbian sexuality is inconceivable under heteropatriarchy. She writes:

> Our desire is boundless. Our Lesbian love does not occur inside boundaries from violation, but within the realm of safety created by connection . . . There are no sexual acts. This desire, this opening between partners is not defined by whose what is rubbing whose whatever when. Any focus on sexual acts or techniques limits our ability to be present to one another. Sex is always relational even when it is solo. There is an infinity of ways Lesbians make love (Hart, 1996, 77).

Seventy-one per cent of lesbians in my sample were in lesbian relationships at the time of completing the questionnaire. One participant indicated that she was in two sexual relationships simultaneously. The length of time women had been in their present relationship varied between two months and 30 years. Of these women, 84 per cent were sexually active with their partners. Lesbians who were not sexually active with their partners wrote of the love and intimacy that they shared and explained this in ways that reflect Nett Hart's contention. For example:

> Genital sex is infrequent, however, I continue to be sensual and intimate with my partner. [73]

> When we met we were bonding beautifully – energetic, orgasmic days and nights. We would hold each other, rock each other and kiss each other, massage, care for and remind each other of our love and sometimes we fuck. Basically fucking is not a priority, however, our love for one another is. [204]

However, some lesbians do not accept that 'real' sex can be anything other than genital sex as is evidenced by the following questionnaire responses:

> We stopped being sexually active four months ago. It just seems to have happened – a different sort of intimacy has

developed. I haven't ruled out sexual activity in the future; just at the moment it feels right. [6]

Similarly another woman remarked:

. . . we have less genital sex now and more moments of quiet, sensual/sexual intimacy. We've probably toned it down some. [28]

And another participant explained:

We never started a sexual relationship. We decided that we would rather have a sensual intimate relationship that focussed on caring and nurturing each other rather than engage in a sexual relationship that might inhibit our creative ways of experiencing sensual intimacy/pleasure. Initially we had both been in heterosexual relationships and needed to overcome social conditioning. This is by far the most connecting and intimate relationship I have had. [142]

These words support Nett Hart's critique of hetero-patriarchal views of sex and illustrate how powerful and pervasive such views are. As Hart asserts:

There is no way the programming we received about sex can be translated into a woman-loving context. We have to invent it, discover it, do it. We only know what we are discovering stroke by stroke, lip to lip, Lesbian to Lesbian (1996, 77).

Clearly, many lesbians in my study were inventing and discovering lesbian sexuality.

Menopausal age or stage?

Many studies have concluded that, in general, sexual activity declines with advancing age. However, there is little, if any, consensus about the cause of this decline. Some authors argue that it is based on biological factors, others on hormonal changes, and yet others on an interaction of a variety of factors including the social context in which women live their lives. A major problem with these studies is that they have mostly been conducted with heterosexual women. As I pointed out earlier, very few studies exploring the relationship between menopause and sexuality have been conducted with lesbians. Results from my study do not necessarily support the notion that sexual activity declines with age. One major problem, in the other studies, I suggest, is the definition of sexual activity. According to mainstream research there is only *one* valid form of sexual activity and that is said to be heterosexual. Therefore, women who do not engage in heterosexual sexual activity are assumed to be celibate.

Nancy Avis and her colleagues (2000) conducted a study to determine if there is an association between menopause status and various aspects of sexual functioning. The sample was taken from a sub-study of the Massachusetts Women's Health Study and consisted of 200 women who were naturally menopausal and not taking HRT. The average age of the women in the sample was 54 years. One-third of the sample was premenopausal, one-quarter perimenopausal and the remainder, postmenopausal.

All of the women in this study had current sexual partners and 89.5 per cent were married. The authors acknowledge the heterosexist bias of their research and make it clear to the reader that their sample included heterosexual women living with a male partner. It is thus not surprising that many of the questions focused around the issue of 'sexual intercourse'. Findings indicated that the postmenopausal women were more likely to believe that sexual interest declines with age and reported decreased arousal. Married women in this study reported a decreased sexual arousal at this time in their lives, compared with when they were in their 40s (2000, 304). The authors point out that their results are consistent with other studies.

In a study from the UK, Keith Hawton and colleagues (1994) found in a randomly selected community sample of women that the age of the woman and her male sexual partner were significant predictors of sexual frequency. This study found that women enjoyed sexual relationships less as they aged and many found it to be 'unpleasant'. Older women commonly preferred less sexual activity. The duration of the sexual relationship also played a role in the level of women's enjoyment in sexual activity. It was found that sexual enjoyment decreased along with the duration of the relationship. The authors suggested that advancing age was associated with increased reporting of sexual dysfunction significantly more than of menopausal status. These findings are consistent with other research results, which also report a decrease in sexual interest, enjoyment and activity with age (Hallstrom & Samuelsson, 1990; Segraves & Segraves, 1995). Perhaps a reason for the decline in sexual activity is closely related to the woman's feelings for her male partner rather than menopausal age or stage. As sexual enjoyment and frequency was found to decrease along with the duration of the relationship, I suggest that rather than conclude that a woman is suffering from sexual dysfunction, a more helpful approach would be to ask her how she feels about her partner. It might transpire that with advancing age comes certain freedom, and heterosexual women may feel less compelled to conform to societal expectations as they grow older. As we will see, many lesbians in my study report that being a lesbian at midlife brings a sense of freedom.

Menopause, marriage and sexual activity

In a more recent study, Phyllis Mansfield and co-researchers (1998) examined the relationship between particular sexual qualities women at midlife desired in themselves and their husbands. The sample consisted of 280 women participating in the US Midlife Women's Health Survey. The authors note that only married women were included, as their previous research (Mansfield et al., 1995) showed that '. . . being married was a significant predictor of certain sexual-response changes' (1998, 289).

Mansfield and her colleagues point out that 60 per cent of the women in the study did not report any changes in their sexual responses over the past year. Of the 40 per cent of women who did report a change, these changes were mostly in declines: in desire, frequency, enjoyment, arousal and ease of orgasm. An interesting and perhaps surprising finding revealed that 'one fifth of the women reported increased desire for non-genital sexual expression e.g. cuddling, hugging, kissing' (1998, 297). The authors suggest three possible explanations for the increased desire for non-genital sexual expression. Firstly, they believe that women may be desiring more non-genital sexual expression in an attempt to 'facilitate their sexual responsive- ness to intercourse, including arousal and passion'. The implication here is that such behaviours may be a precursor toward more fulfilling sexual intercourse. Once again, we can see how only sexual intercourse is regarded as the real thing; anything else is just warming up to the big event! This is reminiscent of past and most probably ongoing ideas that lesbianism is just a passing phase – before women discover the real sexuality – heterosexuality. Another view of Mansfield and colleagues was that older women are seeking more non-genital sexual expression as a means of enhancing 'their feelings of physical and emotional intimacy' with their husbands (1998, 298). The authors thus highlight how physical affection and non-genital intimacy are constantly valued in women's lives and how men and women's expressions of intimacy differ.

Their third explanation suggests that married women at midlife may desire more non-genital forms of sexual expression instead of sexual intercourse. Anecdotal evidence collected by the researchers suggests that these women '. . . are more likely to seek out non-genital sexual expression in order to enhance feelings of intimacy, and that they prefer this form of sexual expression to sexual intercourse.' One woman stated the following: 'Sometimes I feel I could live without sexual inter-course. But, I do enjoy holding one another – embracing, lying in bed together' (1998, 298).

The authors conclude that these findings may reflect the expectations of how women at midlife believe they should be performing sexually rather than expressing their personal sexual preferences. It is suggested that women experiencing decreased sexual responsiveness at midlife may feel guilt and anxiety as they believe their husbands still want, and perhaps they believe deserve, the same level of genital intercourse as before. The following quote from Mansfield's research illustrates the point well: 'I wish my drive matched my husband's. I feel guilty telling him "No" so often. He accepts the answer, but I know he'd enjoy it more frequently' (1998, 299).

This situation, I suggest, is different for lesbians at midlife who might not be so concerned about societal expectations of 'appropriate' sexual behaviour at this stage of their lives. While I reject a biological and/or hormonal link between menopause and sexual identity, I am pleased to report an exciting and unexpected theme was that many women appeared to come out as lesbians around the time of menopause. A number of women spoke of the freedom that midlife brings and the accompanying sense of time for oneself. The following section discusses lesbians' views about sex and sexuality at midlife.

Lesbians and sexuality at menopause

Although I did not ask women if they had been in long-term heterosexual relationships prior to coming out, several participants readily shared this information with me. It was often written on the questionnaire or discussed in the face-to-face interviews. As this was not a standard question, I do not know exactly how many women were previously married and therefore cannot draw any definite conclusions as to how this may have impacted on their sense of self and well-being. The responses, however, do reveal many common themes among women who were previously married and have come out in midlife. Many women spoke of the feeling of having been controlled and not wanting this control any longer. For some of the participants, it appears that menopause or midlife gave them permission to at last do things for themselves. Merle saw it as if she was now grown up and no longer had to 'toe the line'. She explains:

I think I just started feeling that this wasn't what life was all about and there was something missing. I didn't want to be straightjacketed. I didn't want to feel . . . what's the word . . . not oppressed . . . but controlled. So I started feeling that I actually wanted to do more things on my own, even though my husband really disapproved and he didn't like my friends. I didn't really have any friends; most of my friends were our friends, so if I did make a friend, he really didn't like it and I started to think, well, this is ridiculous, I'm a grown-up woman. I'm not a kid any more. I don't have to be controlled by my parents or . . . 'coz my parents were quite strict, so I had a very strict upbringing. I've always felt that I sort of toed the line and I got to the point where I felt I didn't want to toe the line any more and that happened way before I realised I was gay. I did have close friendships with a couple of women, and he really objected to that. It was actually when my daughter was a baby that I started not wanting to be . . . physically not wanting to be close with him any more, which I found really strange, and I couldn't understand why, actually, but it was very soon after Belinda was born, she's the younger one and . . . it's taken a long time. I got to the point where I really and truly just wanted to be on my own and be able to control my life myself, and I think possibly the menopause . . . just going through that time when I . . . I guess I get frustrated really easily . . . clearly in this

49

hot–cold–hot–cold thing you can't tolerate much and I think my tolerance level was really low and we just came to the point where we thought, right, well, look, we'd better split up right now rather than hang on until the kids finish year 12, so we actually split up while my son was in year 12, which was hard on him, but he still did very well. It was very difficult but it *really* was the best time, and I really think if I hadn't been going through that menopausal stage, I probably would've put up with it until later and then done something, but I just got to the point where I *really* had to change my life. [212]

Merle's comments are similar to those found in a unique study of lesbian sex at menopause conducted more than ten years ago by Ellen Cole and Esther Rothblum (1991). In this US study, 41 women with a mean age of 51.5 years were asked about changes in their level of sexual desire and frequency since menopause. All of the women indicated that they were lesbians, except for one who identified as bisexual and two who did not indicate their sexual orientation. Sixteen per cent of women in Cole and Rothblum's study had a hysterectomy and 34 per cent were taking HRT. Over half the lesbians in this sample were in a committed relationship with a partner. The average length of the relationships was 7.28 years. Most of the women's partners were younger and still menstruating.

Women were asked about changes in their level of sexual desire and frequency since menopause. Sixteen lesbians (39 per cent) reported no change in sexual desire since the onset of menopause. Nine lesbians (22 per cent) reported that their desire had decreased and eleven lesbians (27 per cent) stated that their sexual desire had increased since menopause. Nineteen lesbians (46 per cent) indicated that the frequency of sexual activity remained the same since the onset of menopause; six women (15 per cent) noted that sexual activity had increased and eleven lesbians (27 per cent) stated that it had decreased since the onset of menopause (1991, 188).

Thirty-one women (76 per cent) surveyed stated they did not have a problem with sex. The ten women who indicated that they did have a sex problem spoke of vaginal dryness and a longer time taken to reach orgasm since menopause. Many of these women commented that these were 'differences' rather than problems.

The authors note that in general the responses had a 'celebratory quality'. Many of the participants stated that the changes in their sex lives were not necessarily due to menopause, however, related to other factors such as 'the timely mellowing of our relationship (1991, 186). Twelve women (29 per cent) mentioned an increase in the quality of sex since menopause and stated that sex was now better and more fulfilling. Generally the responses were positive, reflective, insightful and honest. The following quotes illustrate the point well:

> Sex is evener since menopause; less emotional up and down. I experience sex more as a part of life now than as an altered state. It's definitely different, but not better or worse (1991, 187).

> All of my sexual experiences with women – even prior to menopause have been *quality* – unlike the same with men, who I must admit that in my twenties and thirties I had more quantity . . . meaning, I was much more promiscuous with men (quantity) versus the quality of sexual intimacy since 1977 exclusively with women. Since menopause, my orgasms (whether from vibrator, self-stimulation or with a partner) happen more quickly and more multiply (1991, 187).

Women were asked if their favourite way of having sex had changed since menopause and only one woman indicated that it had. The authors conclude that current favourite ways to have sex reflect the women's younger adulthood. Women were asked who generally initiates sex and whether this had changed since menopause. Three lesbians out of 37 who answered this question indicated that these patterns had changed. All of the lesbians in this study have had orgasms. Ninety-three per cent of them orgasm when they masturbate and 90 per cent experienced orgasm with a partner. More than half of the women in this study reported no change in orgasms since menopause (56 per cent), 20 per cent had fewer orgasms and 22 per cent stated that they experienced increased orgasms since menopause (1991, 189).

Cole and Rothblum asked respondents to comment on positive changes in their lives, including sexual lives, since menopause. This addition was included in an attempt to correct the 'usual research focus on pathology during menopause' (1991, 190). Responses were interesting, original and varied. Women wrote about a multitude of things including: the enjoyed absence of periods, increased sex and orgasms, being less driven, a greater sense of self-acceptance, coming out as a lesbian, feeling more free, financial and professional security, nothing to prove, kids leaving home and wonderful sex. Only nine lesbians (22 per cent) indicated that there had been no positive changes since menopause.

The authors acknowledge that just as clinical samples reflect a pathological bias, this volunteer sample may reflect a health bias. They warn the reader to be wary of making generalisations to a larger group and point out that perhaps only those satisfied with their lives at midlife would take the trouble to respond and complete a questionnaire. While this may well be the situation, the data obtained from this small sample are nevertheless important and add a new dimension to the existing data on heterosexual women's experiences of sex and sexuality at menopause. Results from my own study support many of the themes from Ellen Cole and Esther Rothblum's study.

The only other study I managed to find that focused entirely on lesbians and menopause was another US study, 'Coming of Age: The Experience of Menopause for Lesbian Women'

(Davis, 1993). In her Masters thesis Heather Davis interviewed seven self-identified lesbians about their experiences of menopause. Lesbians in this study were English-speaking, aged between 40 and 60 years, perimenopausal or no more than three years past their last menstrual period. Women taking HRT were excluded from the study. Participants were recruited through notices in bookstores, a women's centre, a feminist newspaper and word of mouth. The majority of lesbians in this study contradicted the commonly held belief that sexual activity and desire decrease during and after menopause, and several of the lesbians reported an increased desire in sexual activity (1993, 32).

In my own questionnaire I asked lesbians if their interest and/or desire for sex had changed since the onset of their peri/menopause. Almost 53 per cent of participants indicated that their interest/desire had changed. Forty-three per cent of lesbians reported no change in their level of sexual interest and/or desire, and 4.3 per cent of my participants did not answer this question. Following on from this question, participants were also asked if the frequency of sexual activity had changed since the beginning of their peri/menopause. The results obtained are similar to those found in Cole and Rothblum's (1991) study.

Less than half (48 per cent) of lesbians in my study reported a decrease in frequency of sexual activity and 9.4 per cent indicated an increase. Thirty-five per cent indicated that the frequency of sexual activity remained the same while less than 2 per cent reported fluctuations in the frequency of sexual activity. More than 5 per cent of respondents did not answer this question. The biggest variation between Cole and Rothblum's and my own studies in terms of lesbian sex at menopause relates to the decrease in sexual frequency.

Some lesbians in my study had only recently begun to identify as lesbians while others had identified as lesbian all of their lives. The mean number of years women identified as lesbian was 20.7. Only 17 lesbians out of a total of 116 had been lesbians for less than ten years. As in Cole and Rothblum's study, my sample also included lesbians who were surgically, as well as naturally, menopausal and lesbians who were using HRT. Both studies highlight the fact that it may not be menopause that is responsible for the changes in frequency of sexual activity, but other 'external' influences. As discussed earlier, much of the mainstream (heterosexual) literature identifies partner problems as one of the key determinants in women's decreased interest in sex at this stage of their lives. Findings from my own study do not support this view. Women who indicated that their interest/desire in sex had changed since the start of their menopause (52.5 per cent) did not suggest the change was due to partner problems. Partners were identified as a problem only in terms of lesbians who did not have a partner, rather than as sexual difficulties in a partner. The reasons lesbians gave for the decrease in sexual interest and/or frequency, related to external or situational factors rather than reflecting a biological or hormonal basis. These factors included tiredness, lack of energy, stress, tension, length of the relationship, daily stress of managing work and family life and geographical constraints, such as partners living in different states and in some cases, different countries.

I asked participants to complete the following sentence: 'The main factor affecting my sex life at this time of my life is . . .' and responses revealed a variety of factors impacting on this change, very few of which related directly to the menopausal experience. For example, the main factor affecting this study participant's sex life at this time of her life is '. . . the fact that we have a six-year-old son and we are both exhausted by bedtime'. [33]

Or, as another participant put it:

I'd be hard pressed to say that my lack of interest in sex is due to menopause. More likely it is a weighing up of priorities. Do

I want to expend energy fucking then sleeping, like knocking out half a day in a weekend, or do I want to study and work towards making a significant change in making our schools safe places for GLBT[7] kids and teachers? I choose study. I'm just not focussed on sex. [204]

Nevertheless, whilst it was not a common view, some lesbians did see their declining sexual interest directly related to the menopausal process. In response to the question asking them to identify the main factor affecting their sex lives, one woman wrote:

... all due to loss of hormones. HRT does not fully restore sexual function and in my case has caused weight gain that I have gradually adjusted to. I feel very sad for my loss of full sexual enjoyment and function. The desire, sensation and lubrication is 'just' adequate. [35]

Similarly, another woman drew a connection between the role of hormones and sexual interest/activity. She explained:

... the higher the dose of HRT, the greater the desire for sex, hence the more frequent. I try to take the least amount of HRT to alleviate symptoms. I have a greater desire for sex when I put on a new patch. By the end of the week, just prior to patch changing time, my desire wanes. Without HRT I would prefer to go to bed with a good book. My sex life on HRT would only be limited by a lack of a lover! [12]

HRT obviously played a pivotal role in both these women's sexual lives – however, the other participants on HRT did not confirm this view (see also Chapter 4).

Participants were also asked if the type of sex they enjoy had changed and 29 per cent indicated that it had. Questionnaire responses included:

I had a lesbian relationship for four years in my early 20s but still identified as bisexual at that stage. I then had a twenty-year heterosexual relationship, marriage and raised two magnificent daughters but always thought and hoped that one day I would be with a woman again. I became steadily unhappier in my marriage in the second ten years and gradually lost all desire for sex with my ex-husband and eventually couldn't handle it at all. I continued to do it for the peace and security of the family until I was going crazy and had to summon the courage to end the relationship. During my peri-menopause I became a lesbian again – oh joy of joys! I suddenly discovered that I can still feel very strong sexual desire. I thought I may never get wet again . . . so wrong. This is much better sex than has occurred at any stage of my life. My lover is so understanding and she cares so much. [194]

Another woman commented:

I think I am more interested in sex, not less. This might be because I am no longer living with a man. On the other hand, I genuinely feel more sexually alive. Hot flushes seem to bring other 'heat' with them, which is very nice, actually. [217]

Lesbians in this study were clearly discovering their own sexuality and the type of sex enjoyed was personal and varied. While some lesbians were enjoying less genital sex, others were ecstatic about the increased focus on vaginal sex, as evidenced by the following quotation:

. . . yes [the type of sexual activity I enjoy has changed]. There is an increased focus on vaginal sex as I now ejaculate large volumes of fluid at orgasm, increased masturbation and otherwise less-sensitive clitoris and more G-spot sensitivity. Multiple orgasms and longer sessions of sexual activity. [141]

Contrary to this experience, another participant wrote:

. . . it is worth pointing out that sex, especially penetrative sex, is not as frequent. The style of sex has shifted to a more vanilla level. [125]

Other women wrote how the type of sex they enjoy has changed as a result of becoming more familiar with a new partner and sexual inhibitions disappearing. These responses illustrate how the narrow notions of sex, as defined under heteropatriarchy, are foreign and irrelevant to many lesbians. Annie indicated that her experience of menopause had been affected by being a lesbian, and commented that being in a new sexual relationship with another woman helped her enormously during this time. In an interview, Annie expanded on this and explained:

> I just think I was doing menopause big time when I was in a new sexual relationship, and it was incredibly exciting and so I was just so turned on and so sexual, as you are in a new relationship, but I just walked around saying, 'What are all the people talking about? You know, I have absolutely no problems.' And all the stuff about dry vaginas and, you know, low libido, it was so foreign to me. I had absolutely no problem with a dry vagina. If I did have a relationship that was a bit flagging sexually I think it would be very easy to blame menopause. So much of this stuff is in our heads and I think if somebody's got a flagging sexual relationship and you suggest to them that it could be about their hormones, you cling onto that as being a reason. [131]

Annie's insightful comments present a view of sex and menopause that is not commonly discussed. The fact that she was in a new sexual relationship and felt incredibly turned on seems to be at odds with much of the findings from the mainstream (heterosexual) research. Annie was not the only lesbian in my sample to reject the medicalised and heterosexist view of sex for women at menopause. Andie, a lesbian in her 60s, explained in an interview with me how the focus on dry vaginas and decreasing interest in sex with age is simply not true. Andie explains:

Our sex life has been determined by how available we are to males and how they feel about us. Now, when I was a younger dyke, say in my 40s and 50s, when all the old dykes would say how terrific their lives were, and how much freer they felt, and how much fun they were having, and especially when I would hear them say how great sex was, I simply didn't believe them. I thought they were lying to try and give us some hope, a reason to stay alive, or that they were trying to make themselves feel better by exaggerating their joys and their accomplishments. Or that they were trying to stave off some pain by making it seem not so bad to get old, but I thought they were, at best, misguided, and possibly lying. So here I am, at age 61 in two or three days, and I know that they weren't lying. Yes, it's like an apple, you know even if an apple does get dried up, all you have to do is put it in water, and it will be hydrated. The same with our sex. At one point in menopause, due to a combination of physical menopause and having another round of incest memories, I did dry up, metaphorically, just like a dried-up apple, but then when I came to a different part of my life and was re-hydrated by the love and nurture of others, especially a wonderful partner, and my own willingness to open to that, I'm all juicy again. And I mean literally juicy . . . you know, Jill and I make love and there is plenty of vaginal fluid. Now, there can be some physiological reasons, including ageing, that we might have a little less fluid, but it is absolutely simply not true that we dry up; simply not true. Our eyes don't dry up, our saliva doesn't dry up, and our cunts don't dry up . . . it is all part of the same fluid system. [7]

Elizabeth also spoke of the misdirected focus on dry vaginas and the lubrication 'problem'. She lived the first half of her life as a heterosexual woman and thus was able to draw connections between the two vastly different ways of living in this heterosexist world. In a face-to-face interview, Elizabeth discussed this issue with me:

Because I've had sexual experiences as both heterosexual and as a lesbian, I guess sex is different. Because I know my readings indicate that lubrication is an issue. I think it may be more so with penetration than it is with a lesbian relationship. My experiences of a lesbian sexual relationship is much, much, more than penetration. Whereas, that has something to do with it as well, that sexually there hasn't been any issues; whereas perhaps in heterosexual relationships if lubrication does become an issue and sex does become painful and/or their libidos drop, then there's a lot more issues. But again, it is about what your attitude is and that type of thing as well. I do think my experience as a person in a lesbian relationship, as opposed to a heterosexual relationship, intimacy is quite different. Even in my early times in a relationship other than heterosexual relationship, intimacy is quite different. Now whether that's a maturity thing, or being much more aware of who I am sexually, I'm not sure, but certainly, I'm . . . it's a difficult one. If something was to change we'd have to look at it and work it out as well. It's always under the shower [laughter] that's why we have a double shower, I'm sure.

Elizabeth explains from her experience how lesbian sex is much more than penetrative sex. She speaks passionately about intimacy and how this differs in relationships with women as opposed to men. Several participants in my study discussed these differences, and participants who did discuss sex were often critical of the ways sexual activity is promoted and encouraged in the mainstream. Anne shared with me her views on sex since menopause. She explained how since menopause she feels a more mellow and contented person and 'hankering after sex' is not part of her reality. Anne remarked:

. . . we have this pressure that we have to be sexually active and you have to be 'doing it' all the time, and we tend to be given what I see as the end of the spectrum, which is the abnormal behaviour, so if you go off to 'Sexpo',[8] they presume that what is advertised is what we all should be doing. If you see that viewpoint as what sex is all about and sexual interaction, then I see that as one end of the spectrum and quite bizarre. We don't tend to be given . . . what I'd like . . . I mean, if you sat people down and asked . . . found out what is going on, I think you'd find a great range of things that are happening. There are personal differences just like there are . . . you know, hair colour, eye colour or whatever. We all feel differently and respond differently, so I think that the pressure that you have to keep going and doing this serves men's purposes rather than women's. Also, you do find lesbians who pick up on these things and start emulating this strange behaviour and being cool and trendy. I think that's a bit disturbing. Since menopause, sexual activity isn't really something that's in my focus. It's just . . . I do tend to feel more self-contented anyway and I don't really feel that I have to keep up with anybody in that way. It's just that I'm doing what I feel I'm comfortable with, and racing off to a bar to chat somebody up to go and have sex isn't part of it.

Ellen Cole and Esther Rothblum's study was the first to dispel many of the myths associated with lesbians and sex from a sample of healthy lesbians. By deliberately asking many of the same questions in my study, I was able to obtain responses from a larger sample of lesbians at midlife and confirm their positive findings.

Cole and Rothblum noted many differences in responses in their study with lesbians when compared with heterosexual women's answers. They observed that heterosexual women in past research were troubled by 'their deteriorating sexuality, performance pressure and fears of disappointing their partners' (1991, 192). Much of the mainstream research previously discussed in this chapter highlights these issues for heterosexual women. Lesbians who participated in their study, like those in my own study, emphasised the quality of their relationships rather than focusing on their sexual functioning. The authors suggest – and I concur – some possible explanation for the stark differences in the responses might relate to the ways in which lesbians deal with living in a patriarchal and homophobic world where youth and beauty are gloried. They suggest that as lesbians are used to living outside the mainstream, they may be less likely to accept the values associated with those of the mainstream (1991, 192). Results from my own study certainly support these suggestions.

As in Cole and Rothblum's study, I asked participants to explain what lesbian sex was like for them at menopause. I asked lesbians to complete the following question: 'Based on my experience, lesbian sex at menopause is . . .' The vast majority of participants reported positive and healthy responses. Examples of questionnaire responses include:

Beautiful, soft, gentle and loving. [3]

Just as good, no, probably better as I am evolving. [8]

Satisfying and changing in its expression. It requires a sense of respect and mutuality given that partners are at distinct phases in their own physical process. [28]

Fulfilling and loving. [30]

With a long-term partner in a relationship based on mutual respect increasing in intimacy as any other time, where intimacy is physical, mental, emotional and spiritual. [59]

As good as it's always been. I feel awful writing this because I feel I should be more sensitive to changes and that perhaps I ought to have attended to menopause more closely! [210]

In summary, the mainstream menopause literature on sex and sexuality invariably views lesbians with reference to heterosexual orientation and sexual activity. With the exception of the research by Ellen Cole and Esther Rothblum, as well as

Heather Davis, the studies reviewed in this chapter show that lesbians are seldom included in past and current research on women and menopause. In terms of sexual practices and behaviour discussed in research studies and the medical literature, sex is once again defined from a heterosexual viewpoint in which it refers only to sexual intercourse. My study highlights the many problems associated with a culture that embraces a heterosexist view of sex and sexuality. Instead, the lesbian participants in my research offer an alternative, positive approach to that of the medicalised, heterosexual view of sex for women at the time of menopause. As many of their comments reveal, the depictions and expectations of sexual activities, as commonly understood in the dominant hetero-sexual culture, are often unfamiliar and irrelevant concepts for them. Some others, however, do view sex as it is seen in the mainstream, and have difficulty accepting that sexual activities may extend to anything other than genital contact. Never-theless, even for these lesbians, the focus on dry vaginas and painful intercourse, as it is commonly featured in the main-stream menopause literature, is a misdirected and inappropriate focus.

Older lesbians, it appears, are mostly invisible in research on menopause and other health-related issues. Just as earlier studies and medical experiments were carried out on men and the results then applied to women, I believe we are repeating these mistakes by using results gained from heterosexual women's experiences and applying them to all women. Such thinking, I assert, is heterosexist and homophobic and ensures that heterosexuality continues to be seen as the norm. Excluding lesbians' experiences in research projects will also keep many lesbians in the closet. Lesbian invisibility serves to protect the interests of patriarchy as it reinforces the dominant heterosexual culture and prevents many women from stepping outside patriarchal norms and exploring and discovering lesbian sexuality. Sadly, many women will never experience the positive, wild, joyful, and satisfying midlife and beyond that countless lesbians know so well.

As Ellen Cole and Esther Rothblum (1991, 193) concluded:

> It is possible that if all women, lesbian and straight, could be free of heterosexist hangups about sexual functioning and the aging process, if all women were not handicapped by fears of aging, partner expectation and the extolling of youth, there would be many more reports of unchanged or better, more rewarding sex and deeper relationships, in our fifties, sixties and beyond. It is certainly something to celebrate that many lesbians already experience menopause very positively indeed.

It is imperative that all women are aware of this positive, alternative approach to menopause, sexuality and midlife. Zest for life at mid-age is real.

4

Hormone Replacement Therapy

Hormone replacement therapy (HRT) has become a hotly debated topic associated with menopause over the last two decades. At the beginning of the twenty-first century HRT remains a subject of great controversy. As I will discuss at length on pp. 85–96, the findings from the Women's Health Initiative (WHI) highlights the risks associated with routine use of HRT and challenges previously held beliefs about the benefits of HRT. The US-based Women's Health Initiative (WHI) is the largest-ever clinical trial and observational study designed to assess the risks and benefits of a number of primary prevention strategies for preventing cardiovascular disease, breast cancer, colorectal cancer and osteoporosis in healthy postmenopausal women. The 15-year longitudinal study was launched in 1993 by the National Institutes of Health (NIH) and includes more than 161 000 healthy postmenopausal women aged 50 to 79 years (McGowan & Pottern, 2000). The National Women's Health Network, the only US national membership organisation that is devoted to the health of all women, was instrumental in the launch of the WHI. After years of arguing about the need for a large randomised controlled trial to examine the effectiveness or otherwise of HRT, the Network considered it to be a major victory when the NIH embarked on such a trial. The results of the HRT trial confirm the concerns of the Network and show that they were indeed right to be wary of the unsubstantiated claims made by pharmaceutical companies about the supposed benefits of HRT. The Network develops and promotes a critical analysis of health issues from a consumer perspective. It monitors the actions of regulatory and funding bodies, health professions and the industry, and identifies and exposes any abuses within the system. It uses a grass-roots action to effect social change. Since it was founded in 1975, the Network has worked on a range of women's health issues. (For further details, see their website, www.nwhn.org.)

Indeed, much of the current literature on menopause focuses on the issue of HRT. However, as I was doing the literature review for my thesis, I managed to find only one study on HRT that mentioned lesbians. This re-emphasises the point I am making throughout this book: once again, lesbians at midlife remain invisible.

Many lesbians have long been aware of the role medicine plays in the perpetuation of compulsory heterosexuality. Perhaps for this reason lesbians may be less likely to take HRT and other drugs reported to enhance sexual enjoyment, improve libido, keep skin supple and maintain our youthful looks. Presently, however, no information is available on lesbians' usage of these medications, and as a result we do not know if lesbians are more or less likely to use HRT than heterosexual women. My study, one of the first to look at the issue of lesbians and their attitudes towards HRT, provides some new and interesting information.

From the 1940s to the twenty-first century

Hormone Replacement Therapy for menopause has been around for more than half a century in the Western world. The 1940s saw many different oestrogen preparations prescribed for a variety of 'female ailments'. These early preparations contained oestrogen (estrogen) only and were referred to as Estrogen Replacement Therapy (ERT).[1] In 1943 an oestrogen preparation was developed from the urine of pregnant mares. This was manufactured by Ayerst Laboratories and given the brand name of Premarin (*pregnant mares' urine*).

In 1966 Robert Wilson, a prominent Brooklyn-based gynaecologist, published a book, *Feminine Forever*, that espoused his theories of oestrogen replacement therapy. Wilson regarded menopause as a midlife woman's 'deficiency disease' and argued passionately that it could – and indeed should – be treated with female hormones. Wilson believed that women ceased to be feminine after menopause and therefore became undesirable. He claimed that women who used oestrogen looked and felt better, and he began promoting hormone replacement therapy for women from the premenopausal years until the grave (Lewis, 1993). *Feminine Forever* sold more than 100 000 copies in its first seven months, having received much media hype in a diverse range of magazines including *Time* magazine and *Vogue* (Coney, 1993). As I have noted earlier in this book, the entire notion of femininity is highly problematic for many feminists. 'Femininity' has often been used to keep women subservient and subordinate to men. Feminist psychologist, Dee Graham defines femininity as follows:

> Femininity describes a set of behaviours that please men because they communicate a woman's acceptance of her subordinate status. Thus, feminine behaviours are survival strategies. Like hostages who bond to their captors, women bond to men in an attempt to survive, and this is the source of women's strong need for connection with men and of women's love of men (Graham, 1994, xv).

Many lesbian feminists reject the concept of femininity and as a result might be less likely to pursue behaviours and adopt practices that are regarded by mainstream society as reflecting 'femininity'. If femininity is a concept deemed to be of greater importance and/or relevance to heterosexual women than lesbians, it is possible to surmise that lesbians may be less likely to take HRT. However, despite extensive literature searches, with the exception of one study, I was unable to find information that discussed lesbians and HRT use over the past fifty years.

Robert Wilson conducted research and treated women at the Wilson Research Foundation. This organisation received funding from a range of drug companies, including Ayerst Laboratories, the producer of the best-selling menopausal oestrogen product, Premarin. During this time – the late 60s – there was increasing speculation about a possible higher incidence of endometrial (lining of the uterus) cancer among women taking ERT. The first warnings about the risk of ERT and its adverse effects on the lining of the uterus were in fact announced in scientific papers as early as the late 1940s, but in spite of these warnings ERT continued to be prescribed and administered to women during the 1950s and up to the mid 1970s. By 1975, six million American women were regularly taking oestrogen (Coney, 1993, 157).

Earlier claims about the link between ERT and endometrial cancer were finally substantiated in 1975 with the publishing of two articles in the prestigious US and UK medical journals, *New England Journal of Medicine* and *The Lancet*. Not surprisingly, the sales of ERT fell drastically. An information leaflet was prepared by the Food and Drug Administration (FDA), which stated the dangers associated with ERT. The FDA insisted that this information had to be included in all ERT packages. Although the manufacturers of ERT took legal action to ban the insertion of this information, eventually these inserts were made legal in the US. By the late 1980s progesterone was added to the oestrogen and thus a 'new' product was now promoted as 'safe' and 'medically proven' (Klein, 1992, 27).

Today, HRT is commonly administered as two hormones: oestrogen and progesterone.[2] Oestrogen-only therapy is now well established to be associated with endometrial cancer (Dennerstein, 1998). For this reason, progestin was added to oestrogen as it is believed to offset the effect of oestrogen on the endometrium by preventing its overgrowth. For women who have no uterus (for instance, because of a hysterectomy), progesterone is not deemed necessary. However, some international studies have now shown that oestrogen is also associated with an increased incidence of breast cancer and gall bladder disease (Ewertz, 1996).

Australian psychiatrist and chief investigator of the Melbourne Women's Midlife Survey, Lorraine Dennerstein (1998) acknowledges that to date little research has been done on these drugs in relation to midlife women, which makes it difficult to give an accurate analysis of the risks and benefits associated with HRT.

She writes: 'The incidence of heart disease is decreasing; that of breast cancer is increasing. This makes it even more difficult to assess whether HRT will have clear benefits in 15–20 years' time' (Dennerstein, 1998, 27). Much of the HRT information remains confusing and contradictory. While many books have been written on HRT for women, authors either tend to endorse HRT entirely or reject it totally. It is not surprising that many women today, after the release of the WHI study, are confused and concerned about HRT.

Menopause as an illness

The biomedical model of health views health as the absence of disease and illness. This model assumes that medical treatment can restore the body to good health (Naidoo & Wells, 2000). In contrast, the World Health Organisation (WHO) defines health as 'a state of complete physical, mental and social well-being and not merely the absence of disease or infirmity'[3] (WHO, 1946). Unfortunately, a great deal of the literature on menopause and HRT reflects the biomedical model of health.

Given that the WHO defines health as '. . . not merely the absence of disease or infirmity', it is interesting that menopause is defined in the following way:

> The permanent cessation of menstruation due to the loss of ovarian follicular activity. Menstruation ceases when the ovaries no longer produce enough oestrogen to stimulate endometrial shedding (WHO cited in NHMRC booklet, 1996, 1).

In spite of WHOs acknowledgement of the social and political components of health, the above quote defines menopause as an illness, an oestrogen deficiency disease. Not surprisingly, WHO also promoted oestrogen replacement therapy as the cure (Ussher, 1992; Coney, 1993). By first constructing a disease, a market opportunity is then created for a magic cure. As I have already discussed in the previous chapter, this is not the first time a disease has been constructed and a market for a medical cure created. Female Sexual Dysfunction is another such example. The following quotation published in *Maturitas*, the European menopause journal, only a few years ago, highlights this point:

> The gradual deterioration in ovarian function seen during the perimenopause results in a marked reduction in estrogen production and a significant decrease in levels of circulating estrogen. Estrogen replacement therapy (ERT) is designed to increase circulating estrogen levels by replacement hormones, prevent the consequences of long term estrogen deficiency, and treat symptoms associated with the menopause such as hot flushes, night sweats and vaginal atrophy which are a consequence of lower estrogen levels (Palacios, 1999, S2).

ERT as explained in this quote is a cure for these 'symptoms' associated with menopause. Thankfully, this medicalised and disease-oriented view of menopause has been and continues to be heavily criticised.

A discussion of HRT would not be complete without a summary of the medical risks and benefits of HRT therapy. Much of the medical literature on HRT focuses on the consequences of HRT use in relation to specific diseases. The main diseases or medical conditions that have been examined are osteoporosis, endometrial cancer (cancer of the lining of the uterus), breast cancer and cardiovascular (heart) disease. In the next section I will give an overview of the impact of HRT on these diseases and conditions. A review of the literature about these interactions demonstrates conflicting viewpoints.

HRT and 'symptom' control

Women are most commonly prescribed HRT for the management of troublesome 'symptoms' of menopause such as hot flushes and night sweats. I use the word 'symptom' in inverted commas, as a symptom is indicative of a disease, which without doubt menopause is not. The *Australian Oxford Dictionary* defines symptom as: 'a change in the physical or mental condition of a person, regarded as evidence of disease' (1999, 1359). As I strongly reject the concept of menopause as a disease or illness, I cannot accept the disease-orientated terminology that has become commonplace when discussing menopause and other natural life stages and events. But many people now commonly refer to the 'symptoms' of menopause, therefore constructing it as a disease or illness. This disease focus has arguably had enormous benefits for medical experts and pharmaceutical companies. Similarly we often hear about the 'symptoms' of pregnancy. Women and health professionals alike frequently speak of having a pregnancy 'diagnosed'. The insidious use of such medicalised and disease-orientated language is indicative of further medicalisation of women's lives. Such language and approach, I believe, requires constant challenging.

Numerous studies have been conducted and reported that HRT is effective in relieving hot flushes, night sweats, vaginal dryness and urinary problems. Prior to the release of the WHI findings in 2002, it was also believed that HRT protected women against heart disease, and many women were prescribed HRT for this purpose. HRT has also been prescribed to prevent osteoporosis. It is now widely accepted that doctors were wrong in their assumption that heart disease and Alzheimer's[4] could be prevented with HRT.

It is quite true that for some women, the onset of menopause does bring medical problems, and in some cases HRT can indeed alleviate or minimise the distress experienced. The most common 'symptoms' associated with menopause are hot flushes and night sweats. Australian gynaecologist and first President of the Australian (now Australasian) Menopause Society, Barry Wren states that 'symptoms' such as hot flushes, sweats, insomnia and a dry vagina are experienced by 40 to 70 per cent of menopausal women (Wren, 1989, 35). Other researchers have estimated this figure to be as high as 85 per cent (Hammond, 1989; Rebar & Spitzer, 1987). Susan Davis, Director of Research at the Jean Hailes Research Unit, Melbourne, writes of HRT that '. . . no other therapy has been shown to be as effective as oestrogen replacement in reducing hot flushes' (Davis, nd, 1). Complementary (or alternative) therapists, however, dispute this claim.[5]

Despite the fact that many women experience hot flushes, (or flashes as they are called in American-English), for most women these hot spells do not cause severe problems and the majority of women do not seek medical attention for them. While I certainly do not wish to trivialise the difficulties some woman experience at the time of menopause, nor criticise or condemn women who take HRT for relief of their hot flushes, it must be pointed out that not all women experience major problems at this stage of their life.[6] Sociologist and Associate Professor in Public Health, Jeanne Daly, identified in an

Australian study three categories of women going through menopause. She claimed a minority were 'besieged with problems', most 'battled through problems' and the third group 'glided through mid-life'. These findings support the view that menopause is a highly complex individual and socially influenced experience, which extends far beyond the biomedical model (Daly, 1997). Daly's findings highlight the limitations of the biomedical (disease-focussed) model.

Women who do seek medical attention for hot flushes usually present with multiple issues and might be more likely than women among the general population to seek medical intervention in general (Lock, 1991). It appears obvious to me that if such a large percentage of midlife women are experiencing similar changes, then rather than reflecting a disease, these changes reflect a 'normal' or usual transition from perimenopause to postmenopause. Sadly, however, I suggest that the biomedical model does not embrace a healthy approach to such changes.

Many lesbians in my study, although experiencing physiological changes at this time in their lives, did not seek medical intervention. The following quote from a participant explains why she did not consult a health professional:

There seems to be an assumption that a 'change' means a 'problem'. I haven't consulted health providers and have discovered that for me, the changes were a stage on the way to menopause. I believe they would've been 'treated' had I seen a health provider and I'm glad that I did not. But I have found very little useful information when I just want information about how common each change is. What I've found when I looked was that the change would be under a heading such as 'problem' and then of course a 'solution'. I didn't want a solution because I didn't think I had a problem, but I would have liked to assure myself that it was NOT a problem [9].

Women need and deserve accurate information on the changes taking place in their bodies and all of the options available to them. It is only then that we will be in a position to make an informed choice as to what remedies, if any at all, we would like to use, at this stage of our lives.

HRT and cardiovascular disease

Cardiovascular diseases are diseases of the heart, its blood vessels and the veins and arteries throughout the body and the brain. A stroke occurs as the result of a blood flow problem in the brain. It is considered a form of cardiovascular disease. Coronary heart disease is the most common form of heart disease. It involves a reduction in the blood supply to the heart muscle by narrowing or blockage of the coronary arteries. If women are non-smokers and do not have diabetes they rarely develop heart disease prior to menopause (Barrett-Connor, 1996). After menopause, however, coronary heart disease (CHD) is the leading cause of death for women (Grady et al., 1992).

In 2000, 12469 women died from coronary heart disease in Australia. This figure is almost five times as many deaths as from breast cancer (Australian Institute of Health and Welfare, 2000, 44). This trend continues across the globe. In 2001, 248184 women died from CHD in the US. This figure accounts for 49.4 per cent of the total mortality from heart disease. (American Heart Association, 2004). Cardiovascular disease accounts for the death of more Canadians than any other disease. During 1999, 19002 women died in Canada from CHD (Heart and Stroke Foundation Canada, 2004). Cardiovascular disease is the biggest killer in the United Kingdom.

In 2002, 55727 women died from CHD in the UK (www.heartstats.org). While many women all over the world are aware of the risk and extent of breast cancer, most women remain unaware of the prevalence and risks of cardiovascular disease. In the US, the National Heart, Lung and Blood Institute (NHLBI) has developed a national campaign, 'The Heart Truth' to inform women about their risk factors for cardiovascular disease (www.nhlbi.nih.gov/health/hearttruth/whatis/index.htm).

Many early observational studies[7] showed that the risk of coronary heart disease is 35 to 45 per cent lower in post-menopausal women using HRT than in those women not using HRT (Henderson et al., 1991; Stampfer et al., 1991). These studies were based on women taking oestrogen replacement therapy only, e.g. Premarin (National Health and Medical Research Council, 1996, 5). However, as a result of the WHI findings, it is now widely accepted that HRT does not provide any cardiovascular benefit for menopausal women, and as such, HRT should not be prescribed for this reason.

The US Nurses' Health Study and its second-stage follow-up study, the Nurses' Health Study II, are among the largest prospective investigations into the risk factors for chronic major diseases in women. These and other studies have suggested that hormone therapy users may make healthier lifestyle choices than non-users. These healthier behaviours may include better diets and regular exercise, healthier lifestyles in general and thus, it is argued, the positive outcome in these observational studies of women may not be due to the effect of hormones (Vandenbroucke, 1995).

Some early studies suggest that the women most likely to gain the greatest benefit from HRT are those with existing cardiovascular risk factors. The American Heart and Estrogen/progestin Replacement Study (HERS) however, revealed contrary findings. Beverley Vollenhoven, Senior Lecturer in the Department of Obstetrics and Gynaecology at Monash University (Australia) and consultant gynaecologist, sum-marises the study as follows:

This study was a randomised, blinded placebo controlled secondary prevention trial undertaken in 2763 postmenopausal women with coronary disease. These women were administered continuous combined treatment or placebo. The results showed on an average follow up of 4.1 years treatment did not reduce the rate of overall cardiovascular events in these women and did increase the rate of thrombo-embolic events (first year) and gall bladder disease. The treated women had a significantly greater number of coronary events in the first year and fewer in years 4 and 5 (Vollenhoven, 2000, 9).

In this prospective study neither the researchers nor the women actively involved in the trial knew who was receiving the placebo and who was getting the HRT (this is called double blinded, placebo controlled). This type of medical trial is generally regarded as well designed, as it allows little room for health professional bias. Those administering the medication/placebo are not aware of who is receiving the 'real' drug and who is not. In this situation it is less likely that the people who administer the medication may influence the recipient's responses.

The HERS trial showed that in women with existing heart disease who were taking HRT, there was an unexpected excess risk of blood clots in the first year of the study and no overall prevention of heart disease. This trial also demonstrated that there was some harm from HRT to women and no benefit. The researchers concluded that if women were being prescribed oestrogen purely as a means of preventing heart disease then this was simply not appropriate (Barrett-Connor, 1999).

This study received much criticism with HRT proponents focussing on the fact that it did not continue until its planned period of observation (4.1 years versus 4.75 years). It has been suggested if the study had continued, the results may have been different, as there was a trend that suggested a possible late benefit of treatment (Whitehead & Stampfer, 1998). These cries of protest from medical scientists, menopause 'experts' and others are similar to those recently heard following the publication of the WHI study in 2002 and 2004 (see pp. 88, 93).

Clinical recommendations currently state that 'in those with established vascular disease HRT can not be recommended on the basis of existing data' (Teede, 2000, 8). These results support the findings of the WHI that I will discuss later.

Leading US epidemiologist and Professor of Family and Preventative Medicine at University of California, Elizabeth Barrett-Connor (1996), after summarising all the epidemiologic evidence about the link between HRT and cardiovascular disease, concluded that the majority of published reports suggest that the risk for CHD events is reduced by as much as 50 per cent in postmenopausal women who use oestrogen. This paper, however, was published before the WHI results were released. Mary Ellen Rousseau, a certified nurse, midwife and Associate Professor of Nursing points out that most of these earlier observational studies appear to have 'inherent biases, which might affect the interpretation of the results, either exaggerating or minimizing the effects of oestrogen' (1998, 214). The WHI study is the first randomised controlled clinical trial to examine the effect of oestrogen and progestin on the pre-vention of heart disease and hip fractures. The findings of this study challenge previously held beliefs about the benefits of HRT. As a result of the WHI study, it is now known that there is no role for HRT in terms of prevention of cardiovascular disease.

A US study conducted by Stephanie Roberts and her colleagues (2003) compared the risk factors for cardiovascular disease between lesbians and their heterosexual sisters. In this unique study, 324 lesbians aged 40 years and over living in the state of California and their heterosexual sisters closest in age, were compared in terms of risk factors for cardiovascular disease. The results show that when compared with their heterosexual sisters, the lesbians had a significantly higher body mass index, waist circumference and waist-to-hip ratio;

all of which are known to be risk factors for cardiovascular disease. Their findings suggest that lesbians as a group have greater abdominal fat, which places them at a higher risk for cardiovascular disease (2003, 167). The research team recommend that further studies be conducted in lesbians examining other risk factors such as measurement of blood pressure, lipid, cholesterol and fasting glucose levels. Importantly, the researchers point out that if strategies are put in place in an attempt to decrease abdominal fat in lesbians, a lesbian-specific strategy may be needed. This specific strategy needs to take into account reasons that some lesbians may not see themselves as overweight. The authors acknowledge that weight control is often viewed as feminine behaviour and as such may not be regarded as relevant by some lesbians. This study has important implications for those of us committed to improving women's health and wellbeing.

HRT and osteoporosis

The risk of osteoporosis, like heart disease, is increased after menopause. Osteoporosis is a condition that is characterised by a reduction in bone mass so that the bones become brittle and are more prone to breaking. Osteoporosis has become a major health issue for women in their later years and is likely to increase as the population ages. According to an Australian women's health physician, Sheila O'Neill (1995), for the average woman approaching menopause, the lifelong risk of hip fracture is about 15 per cent. Within one year of fracture, the mortality rate is estimated to be between 12 and 20 per cent (Wark, 1996). It has been suggested that up to 50 per cent of survivors of hip fracture experience severe incapacitation, often requiring assistance with activities of daily living for the remainder of their lives (Rousseau, 1998).

The incidence of hip fracture among women taking HRT is reported to be up to 50 per cent less than in women not taking

HRT (Palmer, 1998). The greatest benefit is seen among women who began taking HRT close to the menopause (started within five years of the menopause) and those who are currently using HRT. When HRT is stopped the bone loss continues. A beneficial effect found in the WHI results relates to the incidence of hip fracture among women taking HRT. The WHI findings showed that 10 women per 10000 taking HRT sustained a hip fracture, compared to 15 women per 10000 taking the placebo (Bhavani, 2002). While this finding is undoubtedly pleasing, the overall risks and benefits of HRT must be considered. Prior to the release of the findings of the WHI some researchers suggested that a more effective means of preventing hip fractures is through '. . . lifelong hormone therapy commencing either at the menopause or at age 65 years' (NHMRC, 1996, 8). This extreme suggestion is another example of the increasing medicalisation of women's lives. Surely, more emphasis needs to be placed on prevention of osteoporosis, rather than focusing on treatment. An update by the Australian Drug Evaluation Committee on the TGA website reads:

> In the light of the recent information on long-term effects of HRT, the Committee concluded that the use of HRT for any long-term disease prevention cannot be generally justified as the potential harm may outweigh potential benefits. This concern applies also to the use of HRT to prevent osteoporosis (www.tga.health.gov.au/docs/html/hrtadec2.htm)

The National Women's Health Network (2002) explains that osteoporosis per se is not the problem; rather it is the fractures which might occur as a result, which lead to disability and death. The authors point out that osteoporosis is not a disease; it is one risk factor for bone fractures. There are many risk factors associated with the prevalence of osteoporosis. Diet and lifestyle are known to contribute to osteoporosis. Low calcium intake, cigarette smoking and lack of physical exercise are, according to Sandra Coney, New Zealand feminist, health activist and author, the three major modifiable risk factors for most well women. White women are more likely to develop osteoporosis than women from any other racial group. The exact reasons for this remain unclear. Similarly, women who are of a slight build are more likely to fracture their bones than heavier women. Fat is a protective factor for osteoporosis. Unfortunately, as acknowledged by the National Women's Health Network, women usually only hear the simplistic message that it is menopause which causes osteoporosis and that HRT will prevent or treat this 'disease'.

Sandra Coney argues that it is wrong to simply blame loss of oestrogen for bone fractures experienced by postmenopausal women. She explains that at menopause women tend to lose approximately two per cent of bone mass annually, with the greatest reduction occurring in the first five or six years after menopause. Coney argues that at the age of 65, women's bone loss slows to the same rate as men's, which is approximately 0.2 per cent per year. She suggests that an emphasis needs to be placed on factors that may decrease the risk of falls in old age. These factors, she suggests, include attention to safer living environments and current drug use, especially those that might make women drowsy and hence unstable. Once again, attention is focussed on medical treatment rather than the promotion of healthy diets, behaviours and lifestyles and a reduction of the medicalisation of women's lives.

HRT and endometrial cancer

As was borne out by the heavy use of ERT in the 1960s and 1970s, as discussed earlier, several studies have observed an increase in the risk of endometrial cancer in women with an intact uterus taking oestrogen alone (Judd, 1996; Writing Group for the Postmenopausal Estrogen/Progestin Intervention Trial, 1995). This risk increases substantially with prolonged use (more than ten-fold after more than ten years), and the risk persists for several years after women have stopped taking oestrogen (Grady et al., 1995). However, as with most of the research on hormone replacement and menopause, the literature on the relationship between HRT and endometrial cancer is both confusing and contradictory.

For example, a US reproductive endocrinologist, R Don Gambrell, noted a decrease of 50 per cent in the risk of endometrial cancer compared with women who were not using HRT.

Another study, prior to the WHI, however, reported that women on HRT were at a slightly increased risk of endometrial cancer (Beresford et al., 1997). The confusion and conflicting information makes it extremely difficult for women to decide what to do at menopause. According to the results of the WHI, in the case of endometrial cancer, HRT was found to be as safe as a placebo. Results from the WHI show that HRT decreases the risk of endometrial cancer to one per cent.

HRT and breast cancer

In the case of HRT and its links to breast cancer, we find yet again that the literature is confusing and conflicting. Some studies show a relative increase in the risk of breast cancer among women using HRT, while others show no increased risk (NHMRC, 1996, 10). The WHI findings, however, answer many of the questions relating to breast cancer and HRT use (see pp. 87–8, 93).

Several studies have shown that the risk of developing breast cancer may be related to the duration of HRT use. Graham Colditz, Professor of Epidemiology and Director of the Harvard Center for Cancer Prevention, and his colleagues reported that the risk of breast cancer was significantly increased in women currently using HRT as opposed to postmenopausal women who had never used HRT. And as the duration of use increased, so did the relative risk (Vollenhoven, 2000, 11).

However, an earlier published retrospective study showed contradictory data. A study reported in the *Journal of the American Medical Association* found that the use of HRT for eight or more years was not associated with an increased risk of breast cancer and was instead associated with a reduced risk (Stanford et al., 1995). But these statistics have since been challenged as a result of the WHI findings (see p. 87).

Susan Davis reassures women by stating, 'a recent review of the world literature on 52000 women with breast cancer and 108000 controls found no significant increase in breast cancer in women using HRT for less than five years' (Davis, nd, 2). Davis writes that:

> . . . for women who had used oestrogen replacement therapy with or without progesterone for more than five years, a relative risk of 1.35 was reported. The use of HRT for more than five years had resulted in 2 extra breast cancers being diagnosed in every 1000 users. The use of HRT for about 15 years had resulted in 1 extra cancer being diagnosed in every 100 users.[8]

Of the women who develop breast cancer while taking HRT, studies have reported that they have a better prognosis as their tumours are less advanced (Cobleigh et al., 1994) and that their mortality is decreased. While at some level this appears to be good news, it does, however, highlight another angle of the increasing medicalisation of women's lives. It implies that if a cancer is detected (and as Susan Davis tells us, with HRT use for more than five years, an extra breast cancer is found in every 500 women) it will be found at an earlier stage and therefore treatment will be less invasive and the outcome for the woman more favourable. This fact, I suggest, would bring little comfort to the woman who develops breast cancer as a result of using HRT for five years or longer.

An Australian study by Anne Kavanagh, Heather Mitchell and Graham Giles (2000) found that HRT use reduces the sensitivity of mammographic screening. A mammogram (breast x-ray) provides a picture of the inside of the breast and can detect early breast changes that may constitute breast cancer, even where there are no symptoms. A screening mammogram differs from a diagnostic mammogram. Screening mammograms are performed on women with no symptoms of breast disease to detect breast cancer at an early stage. Screening mammograms are free of charge in Australia through the National Program for the Early Detection of Breast Cancer (BreastScreen) for all women over 40 who do not have breast symptoms. Current research indicates that regular mammography is not as effective in detecting early breast cancer in women less than fifty years of age. For this reason the program specifically targets women aged 50–69 years (www.breastscreen.info.au/health_prof/index.htm).

Diagnostic mammograms are performed on women who have breast symptoms that need to be investigated. If a woman has an existing breast problem then a diagnostic mammogram, rather than a screening mammogram, is needed. This is not part of the BreastScreen[9] program and a doctor's referral is required.

In the study by Kavanagh and her colleagues, the investigators examined the sensitivity, specificity and small cancer detection rate amongst 103770 women in Victoria, Australia who attended BreastScreen for a first screen in 1994 and who did not have a history of breast cancer or breast symptoms at the time of screening. Findings revealed that the sensitivity of screening mammography was lower in women using HRT than in women not using HRT. The BreastScreen program has been criticised for not screening women less than 40 years of age. One of the reasons that younger women are not screened is due to the unreliability of the screening in this age group. The breasts of younger women (prior to menopause) are usually dense because there is more glandular tissue than fatty tissue. After menopause however, the glandular tissue of the breast is usually replaced by fatty tissue. This difference in breast structure changes the appearance of the breast on the mammogram. Combined HRT increases breast density (BreastScreen Queensland, nd). This increased breast density makes it more difficult to differentiate between normal and abnormal breast tissue and thus a small cancer may not be detected. According to an information sheet for general practitioners entitled 'Hormone Replacement Therapy and Screening Mammography', an estimated 10 per cent of combined HRT users have extremely dense breasts (BreastScreen Queensland, nd).

The authors of the Australian study point out that of the women diagnosed with cancer during the two-year screening interval, women using HRT were more likely to have a false negative result than non-users of HRT. In other words, women using HRT were more likely to be recalled and have further invasive investigations in order to determine if the abnormality that was detected on the mammogram was indeed cancer or not. The psychological effects on the women during this stressful time must not be overlooked. Although some of these women were given reassurance that they did not have cancer, for some of these women, this was a false or inaccurate result.

Similarly, of the women who were not diagnosed with cancer during the screening interval, women using HRT were more likely to have a false positive result. For these women who underwent additional invasive procedures and undoubtedly experienced psychological distress, their positive breast cancer diagnosis was inaccurate. Both of these situations illustrate the problems associated with mammography screening and HRT use. The possibility of having a small cancer detected among all of the women screened was lower in the women using HRT. The authors remark that 'an additional 23 cancers or 20% more cancers would have been detected by screening among HRT users if the sensitivity of mammography was the same as for non-users of HRT' (2000, 272). In the year 2000, more than 177000 women attended the BreastScreen Victoria program and of those, 1077 breast cancers were diagnosed (BreastScreen Victoria, 2000, 4). Over one quarter of women attending BreastScreen Victoria in 2000 reported using HRT (25.5 per cent) at the time of screening. Given this information, it appears that women presently using HRT and attending BreastScreen every two years are receiving false reassurance. The fact that HRT reduces the sensitivity of mammographic screening may, according to Anne Kavanagh and colleagues '. . . undermine the capacity of population based mammographic screening programs to reach their potential mortality benefit' (2000, 270). As the majority of women who attend the BreastScreen program are unlikely to ever read medical journals such as *The Lancet*, I suggest they are blissfully unaware that their mammogram is any less sensitive than other women who do not use HRT. While many women are using HRT and attending BreastScreen every two years in the belief that they proactively look after their health, they are, in my opinion, being misled.[10] This increasing reliance on medical technology without knowledge of its limitations – and indeed its aggravations of stress due to fear and anxiety – is hazardous to women's health and wellbeing. I believe this type of information, that is, problems with mammograms, must be available to all women to enable them to make truly informed decisions about their own health.

As a nurse and one who has worked for the BreastScreen program, I was interested to learn if lesbians in my study were more or less likely to use the services of BreastScreen. Studies from the US suggest that lesbians might be less likely to perform breast self-examination, obtain mammograms and undergo clinical breast examinations than heterosexual women (Carroll, 1999). Little is known, however, about the Australian situation, as presently such information is unavailable. Despite some research that suggests the risk of breast cancer in lesbians might be as high as one in three (Haynes, 1994), BreastScreen does not ask questions about a woman's sexual orientation. I wish to point out that it is not the woman's sexual orientation that may put her into a higher risk group; it is that some lesbians may have more risk factors for breast cancer than heterosexual women (see Chapter 5). These risk factors include: higher body mass index, greater rates of alcohol and tobacco use and lower rates of childbirth and breastfeeding (Cochran, 2001).

The Women's Health Initiative (WHI) and other HRT studies

A controversy surrounding HRT was unleashed with the findings of the Women's Health Initiative (WHI) in July 2002 (see page 87).

Despite millions of women worldwide being prescribed HRT, the risks and benefits of postmenopausal hormone replacement therapy had not previously been tested in randomised controlled clinical trials in healthy postmenopausal women (McGowan & Pottern, 2000, 110). A randomised controlled trial is the scientific way of validating a medical treatment as effective. When using this method, people with the same medical condition are randomly divided into two groups. One group receives the medical intervention and the other receives a placebo (dummy pill). These two groups are then compared and evaluated. If the group who received the medical intervention has a significantly improved outcome compared with the other group, then the treatment is regarded as effective (Naidoo & Wills, 2000). Randomised controlled trials (RCTs) are considered as the 'gold standard' in medical research and are recognised as the most convincing study design.

Archibald Leman Cochrane (1972), medical practitioner and pioneer of the randomised controlled trial, argues that very few medical interventions have been properly evaluated using RCTs. Demand for a cure and/or treatment for a particular medical condition or disease may prevent such trials from being carried out. As a result, some medical treatments are used before they have been shown to be effective. HRT is one such example.

The WHI, some parts of which are still continuing, has three major components: a randomised clinical trial, an observational study and a community prevention study. The randomised controlled clinical trial has over 68000 enrolled postmenopausal women between the ages of 50 and 79. The clinical trial has three study components: Hormone Replacement Therapy (HRT), dietary modification, and the role of calcium and vitamin D supplements for the prevention of osteoporosis-related fractures and colorectal cancer (National Institutes of Health, 2002).

The main objective of the randomised clinical trial was to examine the effect of oestrogen plus progestin on the prevention of heart disease and hip fractures. A secondary objective was to assess any associated change in risk factors for breast and colon cancer. On 31 May 2002, the trial arm of the study, which involved 16 608 women with an intact uterus who were taking either oestrogen plus progestin therapy or a placebo, was stopped prematurely after 5.2 years instead of the planned 8.5 years, because women receiving active therapy had an increased risk of invasive breast cancer and major cardiovascular events (Yusuf & Anand, 2002, 357). A major cardiovascular event is defined as a coronary-related death, myocardial infarction, new angina, a stroke or the development of congestive heart failure or peripheral vascular syndrome.

According to the Writing Group of the Women's Health Initiative investigators, the rates of cardiovascular disease events, heart attacks, strokes, blood clots (venous thrombo-embolism) and breast cancer were increased in women taking oestrogen/progestin (combined HRT) compared to those taking placebo or 'dummy' tablets. The following numbers of women affected relate to the number of women per 10000 women each year. For example, 37 women per 10000 women each year taking oestrogen/progestin had a heart attack compared to 30 women per 10000 women each year taking placebo or dummy pills. Similarly, rates of stroke increased to 29 women per 10000 women taking oestrogen/progestin compared to 21 women per 10000 for women taking placebo tablets. The rate of blood clots was more than double (34 women per 10000 taking oestrogen/progestin had blood clots in the legs or lungs, compared to 16 women per 10000 taking placebo tablets). In terms of breast cancer, a 26 per cent increase was noted in women taking HRT. That is, 38 women per 10000 developed breast cancer on oestrogen/progestin, compared to 30 women per 10000 taking placebo tablets.[11]

In addition to these results, the WHI revealed some beneficial effects of HRT. These beneficial effects relate to hip fractures and colon (colorectal) cancer. Ten women per 10000 taking HRT sustained a hip fracture compared to 15 per 10000 taking the placebo. A surprising result was that there was a 37 per cent reduction in colorectal cancer rates. This means that 10 women per 10000 taking HRT developed colorectal cancer compared with 16 women per 10000 taking placebo tablets. Despite these results, however, the researchers determined that over-all the active treatment was causing more harm than good to the research participants and thus this trial arm of this study was prematurely stopped (Bhavnani, 2002).

The media release of these findings caused mayhem amongst many thousands of women worldwide. The news of the discontinuation of the study was publicly released on 10 July 2002 one week prior to an article published in the *Journal of the American Medical Association* (JAMA) on 17 July 2002. In other words, women were urged to see their doctors for information and advice one week before doctors had the opportunity to read the study findings! Newspaper articles, television reports and talk-back radio were full of news about the WHI results. Leading health and medical experts were in high demand to speak – and provide some clear information to the many thousands of women taking HRT who by now were in a state of confusion, anxiety and fear. Conflicting public views about the relevance and significance of the findings abounded, which unfortunately increased women's confusion and anxiety.

Not surprisingly, worldwide sales of HRT dropped dramatically in the months following the release of the WHI findings in July 2002. Figures from the Australian Health Insurance Commission show that prescriptions for HRT have fallen significantly since then, after many years of increased use. From 1998 to June 2002 prescriptions in Australia for Kliogest, a common form of combined HRT, increased by 225 per cent. However, from July 2002 to 2003, its rate of prescriptions fell by more than a third (Bradley, 2004). Similarly, Wyeth Australia, the company that makes Premia (combination HRT) lost between 30 and 40 per cent in sales immediately after the WHI findings were released. It has been reported that 25 per cent of the estimated 600000 Australian women using HRT discontinued their combined HRT (Verghis, 2003, 3).

According to Intercontinental Medical Statistics (IMS) Health, a company that tracks prescription drug use in Canada, the number of prescriptions written for HRT in Canada dropped 7.4 per cent in 2002 compared to 2001. This number then plummeted a further 27 per cent in 2003. In the US this trend continues. According to Wyeth Pharmaceuticals the number of women using Prempro (oestrogen plus progestin) before July 2002 was 3.4 million. By March 2004 this number had fallen to 700000. Similarly, before July 2002, the number of women using oestrogen alone (Premarin) was reported to be 6.4 million and in March 2004 this had dropped to 4 million.

Not surprisingly, scientists and medical experts were quick to point the finger at faults in the study design and methodology once the adverse findings were released in the *Journal of the American Medical Association*. Bhagu Bhavnani, Professor of Obstetrics and Gynaecology at the University of Toronto, wrote in a letter to the editor of the *Journal of Obstetrics and Gynaecology Canada*:

> . . . the premature termination of the HRT (estrogen and progestin) trial after just 5.2 years was not due to a significant increase in breast cancer numbers, as the general public thinks, but because the number of cases of breast cancer had reached a pre-specified number that crossed the designated safety boundary. This safety limit was, for obvious reasons, set low (Bhavnani, 2002, 689).

Bhavnani points out that the average age of the 'healthy women' selected for the randomised control trial on HRT was 63.3 years, and only 33 per cent were between 50 and 59 years. This is, according to Bhavnani, many years older than the age at which most women commence HRT. Bhavnani informs readers that almost 70 per cent of these women were overweight and, of these, half were obese (body mass index ≥30), that over one third were treated for hypertension and only half of the group had never smoked. The author attempts to dismiss the study findings by suggesting that 'perhaps this is an acceptable definition of healthy women in the USA, but it may not be applicable to the rest of the world' (2002, 690). I would argue that while this might not be a 'healthy' group of women, it might nevertheless be the 'norm' for many women of this age group in the Westernised world. Medical experts in Australia and other countries also emphasise these points and share similar concerns and criticisms about the clinical implications of the research findings. I find it interesting that these concerns regarding the characteristics of the women in the sample were not raised until the adverse findings of the study were released. These responses are very similar to those heard earlier following the publication of the results of the HERS study (see pp. 74–5). Once again, experts are reluctant to accept the findings of yet another study that details the risks associated with hormone use.

In Australia an expert committee was convened by the Therapeutic Goods Administration[12] to assess the findings on the safety of the WHI. The committee comprised some of Australia's leading epidemiologists, cardiologists, oncologists and gynaecologists. The committee supported the conclusions of the authors of the WHI and reiterated that HRT should not be used for long-term disease prevention in postmenopausal women, as the benefits of such treatment do not justify the risks. But many published articles suggest that the 'short-term use of HRT for the relief of menopausal symptoms remains a reasonable option', so the reader is left to define for herself what constitutes short-term and long-term use. For example, the Australian Drug Evaluation Committee (ADEC)[13] summary statement on HRT reads:

> Hormone replacement therapy is an effective short-term treatment option for controlling the symptoms of the menopause. For each woman considering use of HRT, it is necessary that the benefits be weighed against the several risks that have been observed, including that of coronary heart disease within one year and breast cancer after one year, of therapy. Hormone replacement therapy should not be used for the long-term prevention of disease (www.tga.health.gov.au/docs/html/hrtadec.htm)

There is no explanation as to what is meant by short and long term. Similarly, the Jean Hailes website reads:

> The Jean Hailes Foundation, an NHMRC Centre of Clinical Research Excellence in women's health, reconfirms that short-term use of hormone therapy for the management of menopause symptoms that unacceptably impair a woman's quality of life remains a reasonable option. However, long term use of hormone therapy for women over 50 years of age is rarely indicated. Each individual woman should weigh up the benefits and risks of hormone therapy in consultation with her

health practitioner (www.jeanhailes.org.au / comment / com_2004_mar3.htm).

Once again the 'short' and 'long' term phrases are used without any clarification as to what this actually means. An article from the National Association of Nurse Practitioners in Women's Health (US) entitled 'Hormone Replacement Therapy: Guidance From the National Association of Nurse Practitioners in Women's Health' does, however, provide an explanation of these terms. 'Short-term' is defined as from one to four years and 'longer-term' is explained as more than four years (www.medscape.com / viewarticle / 439106). I found this article on a large medical database and therefore it is not likely to be read by the majority of women using HRT today.

In sum, in spite of all the negative findings of the Women's Health Initiative study, women are still not receiving the full details of this study and as a result may be putting their health at unnecessary risk.

The ADEC recommended that information about the risks of combined hormone replacement therapy be detailed on product and consumer information[14] and a review be undertaken into the use in Australia of combination hormone replacement therapy in the long-term prevention of osteoporosis (Therapeutic Goods Administration, 2002). At the time of writing (July 2004) the review has not been completed.

Another study, WISDOM (Women's International Study on long Duration Oestrogen after Menopause), was also put on hold in July 2002 as a result of the findings of the WHI. WISDOM was the world's largest HRT study and was designed to examine the long-term effects of HRT. The study was planned to run over 22 years and involve 36000 women internationally. The United Kingdom's Medical Research Council granted $11 million to Adelaide University in 2001, under the direction of Professor Alistair MacLennan, Head of the Department of Obstetrics and Gynaecology, to oversee the

Australian arm of this study. Unlike the WHI study, women in the WISDOM trial were aged between 50 and 69 years, would receive ten years of HRT and then be followed up for another ten years. On October 24, 2002, the funding for WISDOM was withdrawn and consequently the study ceased (The University of Adelaide, 2002).

Further anger and confusion was caused on 28 May 2003 with another article in the *Journal of the American Medical Association* which concluded that '. . . estrogen plus progestin therapy increased the risk for probable dementia in postmenopausal women aged 65 years or older' (Shumaker et al., 2003, 2651). The Women's Health Initiative Memory Study (WHIMS) was a sub-study of the WHI study and looked at the effects of combined oestrogen with progestin, commonly known as combined HRT, on the incidence of dementia and memory impairment in postmenopausal women older than 65 years. The results showed that 61 women out of 4532 in the study were diagnosed with probable dementia. Of these women, 40 (66 per cent) were receiving the oestrogen plus progestin, compared to 21 (34 per cent) in the placebo group. These findings support those of the earlier study that the risk of long-term usage of combined HRT outweighs the benefits. Despite these results, the oestrogen-alone part of the study was allowed to continue.

Once again, doctors and scientists were refuting the dementia results by questioning the study design, age of the participants and type of hormone combination used. An example of this is illustrated in the following quote found on the Jean Hailes website. Associate Professor Susan Davis, referring to the WHIMS study and Women's Health Initiative (WHI) trial investigating the effects of combined oral oestrogen and progestin therapy in postmenopausal women, informed women that:

> The new information is important but very specific to the type of hormone therapy used and cannot necessarily be applied to

the use of oestrogen alone, non oral hormone therapy or other oral therapies. The findings reported in these manuscripts also cannot be extrapolated to the more conventional initiation of hormone therapy around the time of menopause for symptom relief. On the balance of evidence combined oral hormone therapy should not be initiated in the older woman with the view to prevention of dementia (www.jeanhailes.org.au/comment/com_may27_2003.htm).

In March 2004, yet another arm of the WHI study[15] was stopped prematurely. This oestrogen-only arm of the study followed 11000 women for seven years and was due to continue for another year. Study participants were randomly assigned to a daily dose of either oestrogen (conjugated equine oestrogen – Premarin) or a placebo (dummy pill). As only women who have had a hysterectomy can safely take oestrogen alone (as it increases the risk of uterine cancer in women who have an intact uterus), I have trouble understanding why this arm of the WHI was allowed to run in the first place. This oestrogen-only study aimed to assess the effect of long-term use of HRT in healthy postmenopausal women on the prevention of heart disease and hip fracture and any associated change in the risk of breast cancer. It did not aim to evaluate the short-term risks and benefits of hormones for the treatment of moderate to severe menopausal symptoms (www.nih.gov/news/pr/mar2004/nhlbi-02.htm).

This part of the study found that oestrogen alone did not increase a woman's risk of breast cancer. The added risk is conferred by progestin. However, oestrogen alone did increase the risk of stroke and possibly dementia.[16] The National Institutes of Health (NIH), the US government agency that conducted the study, posted letters to more than 11 000 study participants advising them to stop taking their pills, based on the information they had collected from an average follow-up of nearly seven years, which showed an increased risk of stroke in women aged over 60 years (Stagg Elliot, 2004). Some of the key findings of the oestrogen-alone study include:

- oestrogen alone had no effect (good or bad) on heart disease;
- oestrogen alone did increase the risk of stroke at the same rate as combined HRT does, i.e. an increase of 8 strokes per 10 000 women per year in those taking HRT;
- oestrogen alone did not increase the risk of breast cancer, however, it did decrease the risk of hip fracture.

The NIH conclude that:

> . . . an increased risk of stroke is not acceptable in healthy women in a research study. This is especially true if estrogen alone does not affect heart disease, as appears to be the case in the current study (www.nih.gov/news/pr/mar2004/nhlbi-02.htm).

The WHI research team plans to follow up with the participants from the WHIMS study in an attempt to learn whether the increased risk for dementia continues after the treatment has stopped.

Barbara Alving, Director of the Women's Health Initiative and Acting Director of the National Heart, Lung, and Blood Institute advises postmenopausal women who use HRT or are considering using oestrogen alone or combined HRT to discuss the risks and benefits with their doctors. She states:

> These products are approved therapies for relief from moderate to severe hot flashes and symptoms of vulvar and vaginal atrophy. Although hormone therapy is effective for the prevention of postmenopausal osteoporosis, therapy should only be considered for women at significant risk of osteoporosis who cannot take non-estrogen medications. The FDA recommends that estrogens and progestins should be used at the lowest doses for the shortest duration needed to achieve treatment goals. (www.nih.gov/news/pr/mar2004/nhlbi-02.htm).

In conclusion, more than two years after the publication of the first WHI study's results, many women remain confused and ambivalent about the risks and benefits of HRT. Anna Day, an Associate Professor in the Departments of Medicine and Health Administration at the University of Toronto, explains how women are targeted to receive therapies and treatments to enhance or maintain their physical appearance, even in the absence of adequate studies of the risks and benefits of these treatments (2002, 362). Day cites examples of women being prescribed drugs that produce anorexia and are known to have a significant risk of pulmonary hypertension as an acceptable form of treatment, because obese women are at increased levels of risk of heart disease and diabetes. Similarly, she cites the case of increasing numbers of women being prescribed antidepressants with little knowledge of the long-term effects of such drugs.[17]

Day reminds readers that socio-cultural norms and values of a society in which women and their health practitioner live, influence patient care. As she puts it:

> . . . on the basis of a belief that hormones are associated with youth and health, hormone replacement therapy for women was believed to be good. The WHI has clearly demonstrated that it is imperative that trials assessing the overall risk and benefit of primary prevention interventions for both men and women be conducted before such therapies are broadly instituted. The WHI demonstrates the potential for doing harm . . . we cannot continue to do so. (Day, 2002, 362).

While many within the medical profession and scientific community may continue to criticise the WHI study design, clearly the results have had an impact on both doctors and the women who consult them for information, advice and treatment. The WHI has provided the best available data on the risks and benefits of HRT for menopausal women. We now know that HRT should not be used for long-term preventative effects as the risks clearly outweigh the benefits. We also now know how wrong doctors and scientists were to promote compliance with these drugs in the absence of sufficient reliable data. Perhaps it is time to decisively shift the focus of attention to non-pharmaceutical agents aimed at the prevention of heart disease and osteoporosis, such as smoking cessation programs, exercise regimes, strength training, and healthy eating patterns.[18] As a result of the publication of the WHI findings and the ensuing controversy, many more women are now questioning if there is a place for HRT in 'treating' a natural stage of life. These questions and conversations between women, as well as between women and their doctors, should be regarded as a positive outcome from the WHI. It is important that these discussions continue not only within the medical and scientific community, but also within the wider general community. As my research has clearly shown, if the discussion is limited to the 'experts', then those of us who are invisible within this society will continue to remain unseen and unheard. After all, lesbians, as well as heterosexual women, experience menopause.

HRT and women's 'choice'

Women's attitudes, knowledge and experiences of HRT vary widely. There can be little doubt that women in the Westernised world today are being inundated with conflicting information about this form of treatment. Women have to decide whether to use HRT or not, and in some cases are made to feel that it is the only responsible course of action to take. Christiane Northrup, an obstetrician/gynaecologist and women's health advocate, highlights how women are routinely warned by their doctors of the risks of *not* using ERT (and now HRT), and thus they believe osteoporosis and heart disease are unavoidable without it. With advice such as this, what 'choice' does a woman have? Christiane Northrup explains:

The rare woman who wants to get through menopause *without* estrogen replacement now has to fear that she may not be making the right choice. She doesn't get the cultural seal of approval that she would if she were on ERT.[19] Women may feel better on ERT in part because they are doing the culturally approved 'right thing'. This can be comforting and health enhancing in and out of itself (1994, 465).

In a qualitative study conducted by Myra Hunter and colleagues (1997), women identified three main themes in relation to decisions about their own HRT use. Firstly, they were more likely to want HRT if they were experiencing problematic vasomotor 'symptoms' such as hot flushes and night sweats. Secondly, the doctor's opinion was an important factor in their decision-making process. The third theme identified by the authors related to views and opinions about hormonal medication. Women were concerned about adverse effects and possible health risks, and many questioned whether it was 'natural' to take medication for menopause and were concerned about the fact that it could distort '. . . the natural rhythms of their cycles' (1997, 1545). These findings support the findings of another study which revealed that women who disliked medication were prepared to use HRT because it relieved severe symptoms and was perceived as the means to '. . . a real need to keep themselves well' (Griffiths, 1999, 473).[20] In this study, the 'choice' to take or reject HRT was restricted by varying factors. The reasons women gave included serious health problems; as well as fear and social attitudes, which all contributed to reducing control over their 'choice'.

It is often assumed that with increased information and education women will increase their uptake of and compliance with HRT. While there is some evidence to support this view, an explanation based on education alone is regarded as too simplistic in terms of understanding women's views on HRT (Hunter et al., 1997). Frances Griffiths, a senior clinical lecturer at the University of Warwick, notes that the sense of control a woman feels could be both increased or decreased by information.

An Australian study challenged the idea that active information seekers have a better understanding of the menopause than the general population. In this study, two groups of midlife women, one a group of women who attended menopause seminars, and another chosen at random, were asked to select from a list of 39 changes those they believed to be directly caused by menopause. The study did not mention sexual orientation and yet again a heterosexual orientation is taken as the norm.

The researchers found no significant differences in the commonly available knowledge, or level of biomedical knowledge, between these two different groups of women. The findings indicated that women may well be rejecting a biomedical model of menopause but nevertheless use HRT for many reasons, not just oestrogen deficiency. Other reasons for the use of HRT might include mood swings, depression, anxiety, irritability, loss of concentration, memory problems and muscular pain and stiffness (Fox-Young et al., 1999).

Knowledge of HRT was high among participants in my study. All of the women had heard of HRT and most described it as a combination of two hormones: oestrogen and progesterone. Questionnaire data revealed that women learnt of HRT from a range of sources including lesbian conferences, gatherings and festivals, women's health services, books, printed information, lesbian and women's magazines, as well as through more conventional means such as medical services and health professionals. As mentioned earlier, some research suggests that women will be more likely to use HRT if they have more information about it and a higher level of education. The results of my study do not support this view. Of the 19 lesbians who were using HRT, the reasons they gave for its use were in line with those published in larger studies. Women who were taking HRT stated that it helped with 'troublesome symptoms'. Several indicated that they were advised to go on HRT by their GPs. Other women taking HRT indicated that it helped the discomfort they experienced and they believed it would provide some protection against heart disease and/or osteoporosis. One participant has contacted me since the release of the 2002 Women's Health Initiative findings and reported that she has discontinued HRT as a result of these findings. As previously stated, it must be noted that the questionnaires and the majority of the interviews were completed prior to the publication of the WHI results. Consequently, I do not know if the study's participants have continued or discontinued HRT. When asked, 'What is HRT?', women who were using it often described it in very 'medical' language. This medicalised definition reflects the model of menopause which dominates public discussion in Westernised countries. The following quote from a participant who is not a health professional, but who works in a medical environment and has been taking HRT since 1990, illustrates this point well:

> HRT substitutes equine hormones as oestrogen replacement and, combined with progesterone, protects against osteoporosis and possibly heart disease and ovarian cancer. It aids in protection of bone density when combined with dietary and physical exercise. [105]

In other quotes HRT users also defined HRT in medical language. This is not surprising, given the high number of health professionals in my study, and the fact that popular knowledge of HRT is high among women in the general community. Nevertheless, it is an interesting finding that although a high number (almost 40 per cent) of my study participants are employed in health-related occupations, the overall number of women using HRT in this study is lower than in other studies. Every woman in my study had heard of HRT and, similarly, all were able to explain HRT in their own words. Popular knowledge of HRT reflects a medical understanding of the drug, as is evident from a diverse range of sources including women's magazines, talk-back radio, television programs and newspaper articles. Three of the six participants quoted below are (or were) registered nurses [35, 134, 202]. The following quotes illustrate the ubiquitous medicalised language:

- HRT replaces diminished or ceased supply of oestrogen and testosterone. [202]

- HRT replaces oestrogens and progesterones that are no longer produced by the ovaries. It also aids with treatment of osteoporosis. [164]

- Replaces ovarian hormones at a level sufficient to maintain premenopausal hormonal influence on total body systems and functions. It may cause some women to menstruate again. [134]

- Gets rid of hot flushes and stands a chance of kick starting my menstrual cycle. [125]

- Relieves the symptoms of menopause – hot flushes etc. It also helps protects against osteoporosis and heart disease. It replaces lost hormones. [57]

- HRT decreases calcium loss, prevents hot flushes, slows skin ageing, preserves perineal muscle tone, prevents complete loss of libido, causes weight gain. [35]

In addition to commenting on HRT as alleviating the physical 'symptoms' of menopause, other participants wrote and spoke of emotional and psychological distress experienced at this time. For some women, these feelings were far more distressing than any of the physical 'ailments' often highlighted in discussions of menopause. Pat explained how suddenly she found herself crying and becoming upset at trivial things. This caused her an enormous degree of distress:

Being out of control with my emotions really upset my works. So off I went to the doctor which I'd been to many times but just decided to do nothing, and I said, 'Look, all the other things I can handle, but I can't handle this. I need some help here,' and to my surprise, this doctor had said to me, 'There is something we can do about it. These are your options.' One of them was HRT. She gave me a video and said, 'Go home and watch the video and see what you think. I feel that it will help level out those things and get you back on the right track but that is my opinion. I don't want you doing something that is against what you think. Go home, read up about what different options I've given you,' and some of them were natural things, although there wasn't a great deal on that then, because it was an up and . . . umm . . . new thing even in the shops, you know, health food shops and that; they didn't have as many things as they do now. So I went home, watched the video, talked about it with my partner who I was not . . . (laugh) she was, you know, my 'best' friend then, right? So I talked with her about it and . . . eventually decided, well I couldn't handle these outbursts of being out of control because that wasn't me. So I went back and said, 'I'd like to give it a go,' and she said to me, 'Well, you can stop it any time.' She did also explain to me, as did the video, that there were other things which at that point in time they thought were really good like the reduced risk of osteoporosis and heart disease, but you had to keep an eye on things like breast cancer and . . . so I think she informed me really well and I made my decision on that and decided to try it. Yes, it has helped, absolutely. [174]

Pat is 53 years old, post-menopausal and at the time of the interview (April 2002) had been taking HRT for eight years. Pat told me she was not concerned about side effects such as breast cancer, because she has had both her breasts removed for 'pre-cancerous cysts'. [21] Pat says that as long as she has her Pap tests regularly, she believes 'the benefits [of HRT] outweighed the risks'.

Other women also described 'mood swings' as one of the most difficult and unexpected aspects of menopause. As one study participant put it rather dramatically:

HRT stops me wanting to cry and/or the almost irresistible urge to kill people! [202]

Another woman commented:

I was diagnosed with depression during this time and now, on reflection, I think it was a menopausal symptom, but the link wasn't made at the time [6].

In contrast to these findings, however, the majority of participants expressed views that were antithetical to the medical model view of HRT. This is evident in the following questionnaire responses:

HRT keeps drug companies in business, causes breast cancer, causes diabetes and relieves some symptoms in some women at an unknown long-term cost. [43]

HRT enriches the drug companies and medical doctors. [66]

HRT suspends menopause until such time as HRT stops so it becomes a lifetime prescription unless a woman decides to proceed with her menopause. [73]

HRT enables doctors to give something to older women, whatever the health complaint may be. [154]

HRT puts unacceptable artificial hormones into the body and provides dollars for the industry aiming to medicalise all natural bodily functions. It increases the risk of further illness and cancer but is promoted as preventing heart disease, osteoporosis and symptoms of menopause. It turns women into guinea pigs. [81]

One of the study participants who is a medical practitioner wrote:

As a medical practitioner I do feel it [menopause] has been overly medicalised as a really lucrative business. I do believe HRT and alternative therapies have a significant role to play. As my hot flushes became more severe despite Black Cohosh and soymilk, I am increasingly tempted. [141]

Other lesbians appeared to reflect a more philosophical view of menopause and the role of HRT. For example, Elizabeth, a 47-year-old lesbian explained:

I've always seen it [menopause] as just another life stage, and because I see it as a life stage it's just . . . well, that's just what happens and there will be some inconvenient times and there may be times when you're not feeling very well, but you just get on with it. Lots of women I know have gone and sought medical treatment and some are using HRT, but they are still experiencing what I would have called 'indicators' of menopause. I played sport for a lot of years and you just play with injuries, so things that are inconvenient, like you still swim if you've got your period, 'coz you can't allow . . . or for me, I can't allow issues around menopause or anything like that to get in the way of my life. So I guess it's an attitude towards it that . . . I guess it's like when people have chemotherapy. They either make a decision that it is going to be horrible, horrible, horrible and they put themselves to bed, or they say, 'I have to have this treatment but then I come out and I go back to work and get on with it.' [168]

Prevalence of HRT use

It is extremely difficult to determine the exact number of women using HRT at any given time. It has been estimated that in the state of Victoria, Australia, in the late 1990s, one in four menopausal women was taking HRT (Vollenhoven, 1999). Diane Palmer, Head of the Menopause Clinic at the Royal

Women's Hospital Melbourne, Australia, estimates that HRT is used by 40 per cent of Australian women aged between 45 and 64 years. The ongoing Melbourne Women's Midlife Health Study (Dennerstein et al., 1994) is a longitudinal study which has been following the lives and health of 357 women for more than nine years. Out of the women participating in the study, 42 per cent had tried HRT and 62 per cent were taking HRT in 1994. This figure is very high compared with other countries (Guthrie, 1999).

Sixteen per cent of lesbians in my study were taking HRT at the time of completing the questionnaire in 2001 (n = 19). This number appears to be smaller than the figures cited in other, larger studies. As already stated, it must be noted that the vast majority of questionnaires were completed and returned prior to the WHI research findings being released in 2002.

Almost 14 per cent of lesbians in this sample had previously tried HRT for various durations. Many of these women discontinued its use after a short time. This concurs with the findings of other published studies which show that HRT treatment is frequently abandoned during the first year. Reasons cited for its discontinuation in my study were similar to those cited in other studies by heterosexual women and included concern about the increased risk of cancer, unwillingness to take 'unnatural therapies', unknown long-term side effects, and the fact that for some women, the menopause 'symptoms' persisted despite HRT.

The mean number of years the women involved in my study had been taking HRT was 4.97. Eight out of 18 participants had been taking HRT for five years or longer (two women took HRT for more than 10 years; one woman did not answer this part of the question). Given the 2002 WHI findings, such long-term use could have serious health implications for these lesbians. Clearly, the 19 lesbians taking HRT in my study were well aware of the controversial nature of this medication, yet they stated they believed that they were making informed choices to take HRT.

The Women's Health Australia study data for the Phase 2 survey of the mid-age cohort (47–52 years) found that 23.2 per cent of women were currently taking HRT and 76.8 per cent were not (Women's Health Australia, 2002, 9). The lower numbers of women taking HRT in my study require further exploration and discussion. While I realise that mine is not a representative sample of lesbians living in Australia, therefore absolute conclusions cannot be drawn, I believe it is an interesting finding that the number of lesbians taking HRT is considerably lower than in other studies with predominantly heterosexual women. Some of my study participants suggested that HRT may be more popular with heterosexual women, and several spoke of the role HRT plays in perpetuating the role of 'compulsory heterosexuality'. These comments were reported in both the questionnaires as well as the interviews. Questionnaire responses included:

> I suspect that HRT would be more popular with heterosexual women, maybe because of pressure from their male partner to 'get better quickly' but that is just a thought without any basis in reality. [113]

Although this participant stated that this was 'just a thought without any basis in reality', it appears that for some women the connection between HRT and heterosexuality is very real. For example, Merle wrote that if she were still married she would most likely be taking HRT. Merle is 50 years of age, identifies herself as postmenopausal and had been in a hetero-sexual marriage for 20 years. She has two adult children and has recently come out as a lesbian. In the follow-up interview Merle explained:

> Yes, I suppose it is my own personal experience, but when you are with a man you sort of have to come up to a certain standard,

and the thing is, he would probably encourage me to do something about it [menopause]. Because if I'm uncomfortable then of course I didn't want sex, and that was a big thing. So he'd be encouraging me to take something to lessen the symptoms to make me more comfortable so I'd be happier sort of . . . to go along with whatever he wanted, and yet, with another woman I don't feel that at all. It's sort of like it's normal life, if you're a married woman and your kids are growing up, you're going through menopause, you take HRT. Life is different now and I just don't want to go down that track. [212]

Merle's explanation is similar to the view expressed by Germaine Greer. In *The Change* (1991), Greer explains how HRT is given to women to promote marital sex. Greer cites an earlier study reported in the *British Medical Journal* (Ballinger, 1975) in which only 114 women out of a sample of 539, aged between 40 and 55 years, would discuss sex with the author. In this study, only 40 per cent of the women with poor libido had a good relationship with their husband, compared to 66 per cent of those with unimpaired libido. Greer asserts that these figures are seen to present a case for hormone replacement therapy. She points out that nobody ever asks the woman if her husband is attractive or even a good lover. She writes:

> . . . the wife has already been told how to dress, how to suggest new adventurousness in sex, how oestrogen will make her breasts taut and so forth. Nobody has ever suggested that her problem might be lack of interest. Hers too might be a dull mind, a dull job or a dull husband. Yet people whose minds are not stimulated are likely to have dull minds; housework is a dull job and the kinds of jobs generally done by women outside the home are dull jobs, and husbands can be very dull, especially if their best efforts have already been expended on people they consider more important in their workplace or their playplace. The situation is as unendurable and deadly for a woman as it

is for a man and she should not be encouraged to dose herself with steroids rather than put an end to it (Greer, 1991, 359).

Many interview participants confirmed Greer's notion of HRT and the role they believe it plays in keeping women sexually available to men. Questionnaire data, too, showed similar views on this topic, as is evidenced in the following comments:

HRT provides artificial oestrogen to keep the body younger and sexually available to men. Add progesterone to the recipe to reduce dangerous 'side effects' such as cancer – breast in particular. [59]

HRT may offset symptoms of menopause but I believe menopause is simply delayed. There does seem to be a suggestion in advertising that ageing is delayed, therefore women will be more attractive to men. Taking HRT may turn out to be one of the biggest social drug experiments against women. [72]

Sandra Coney in *The Menopause Industry* argues that the success of the HRT campaigns is largely due to society's obsession with the desire for eternal youth and beauty. She explains (1993, 163):

The appeal through the lay media worked on women's fears about ageing. Women were promised the preservation of their youthful appearance; a powerful inducement in a culture that worships feminine sexual attractiveness. The critique of the postmenopausal woman offered by these doctors and repeated in the lay media – the anxious, wrinkled, depressive – hit a nerve in women's psyche. For many women, their 'looks' were their greatest asset.

Could it be that these messages are internalised to a greater degree by heterosexual women than lesbians? Another lesbian I interviewed spoke of similar issues. Andie asks:

We don't give adolescents something to prevent puberty so why would we give something at the other end to prevent that? What it prevents is what the patriarchal society says we are supposed to continue in. We are supposed to stay sexually available to men, our breasts are supposed to stay firm. We are supposed to be available for servicing men at any moment and menopause takes us out of that realm. So if they delay or prevent menopause, it keeps us their creatures longer. I don't know, what is HRT supposed to do? Supposed to keep us youthful and appealing, with firm breasts and non-ageing skin? HRT is designed to continue the availability of women to men as men define it and our own natural bodies have times when we are not suited for sexual activity with men, if that's our choice. The availability to men is no longer an issue, because we are now the crones. Now we are menopausal and now is the time when we are available to ourselves. And HRT and all of this patriarchal 'when you are an old lady you are useless,' are designed to deny us time for ourselves and each other. Still we manage. [7]

Alistair MacLennan and his team (1995) reported the findings of a study to discover the prevalence of the use of oestrogen therapy in South Australia. One thousand and forty-seven women over the age of 40 were interviewed. The results indicated the then-current use of oestrogen therapy to be 13.6 per cent and those who had ever used it was 24.3 per cent. Many past users had stopped therapy within six months, frequently because of side-effects. The most common reasons cited for taking oestrogen therapy were to relieve menopausal symptoms, post-hysterectomy and to prevent osteoporosis. Reasons for not embarking on oestrogen therapy included women being pre-menopausal, asymptomatic, or being unaware of the therapy. The authors concluded that among current users there is a perception of only short-term benefits. They also believe that misinformation about the therapy exists amongst non-users.

These findings are consistent with another Australian study. As part of the Melbourne Women's Midlife Health Project, in 1991 telephone interviews were completed with 1897 randomly chosen Australian-born women living in Melbourne, aged 45 to 55 years.[22] Sexual orientation was originally asked for, however, the number of women who identified as lesbian was extremely small (Guthrie, 1999). I have not seen sexual orientation discussed in any of the subsequent publications arising from this study.

Twenty-one per cent of the women surveyed by the Melbourne Women's Midlife Health Project were using HRT and most women reported some benefit from HRT. The most commonly reported benefit was the relief of hot flushes. As in other studies, prevalence of HRT use was higher in women over 50 years of age (Shelley et al., 1995). Both Australian studies suggest higher HRT use than in other countries.

The use of HRT varies greatly from country to country and depends on other factors such as age, socio-economic status, social and cultural background and the availability of medical services. White professional women who are highly educated were more likely to have used, or be using, HRT (MacLennan et al., 1995). A number of studies also report that HRT usage is high among the medical population and the spouses of medical practitioners – therefore all referring to heterosexual women.

A study undertaken in Britain to determine female doctors' uptake and experiences of HRT revealed that 55 per cent of women doctors aged 45 to 65 years without regular menstruation had at some point used HRT. Of these, 70 per cent were still taking HRT five years after starting therapy, and 48 per cent 10 years after beginning therapy (Isaacs et al., 1997). The authors conclude that the high usage of HRT by the women doctors reflects the fact that many started the therapy on their own initiative and with long-term prevention in mind. They acknowledge that HRT users may differ in their health-related behaviours from non-users, and that many women may never take up HRT until the benefit-risk ratio is more clearly established.

A Swedish study reported current HRT use to be 88 per cent among postmenopausal gynaecologists and 72 per cent of female general practitioners (Andersson et al., 1998). An American study was conducted to determine whether physicians' beliefs about the risks and benefits of HRT differ depending on their gender or specialty in a managed care facility. The findings reported that gynaecologists were less concerned about the potential risk of HRT on breast cancer and thrombo-embolic events compared with family physicians and interns. Female providers from these three categories differed significantly from their male colleagues in their beliefs about the benefits of HRT in relation to the reduction in risk of heart disease, osteoporosis and Alzheimer's disease. Female physicians were more concerned about the risks of breast cancer than their male colleagues. The researchers concluded that this difference may affect provider–patient discussions about HRT (Exline et al., 1998). Again the participants' sexuality was not queried; heterosexuality as the norm is assumed.

HRT is big business

Sandra Coney in *The Menopause Industry* has comprehensively discussed how HRT has become a huge industry. Pharmaceutical companies are consistently bringing new products onto the market for menopausal women. Presently a wide variety of delivery systems are available for HRT. HRT is now available in pills (slow-release tablets), patches (transdermal), subcutaneous (under the skin), intramuscular injection and even transvaginal administration. In order to increase the popularity and therefore use of HRT, pharmaceutical companies realise that it must be appealing to women and easy to use. In 2003, a year after the publication of the WHI results, there were 3.1 million fewer HRT prescriptions dispensed in Canada than in the previous year. This drop represents a fall of 26.8 per cent (www.imshealthcanada.com/htmen/3_1_37.htm). Although use of all types of HRT dropped significantly in 2003, in Canada, the Intercontinental Medical Statistics (IMS) states that the recently introduced combination oestrogen/progestin skin patch fell at a slower rate, therefore indicating a preference by doctors and women for the convenience of the newer hormonal therapies. Trials are currently underway in Melbourne, Australia, with testosterone in the forms of gel, nasal sprays and patches in an attempt to evaluate the effects of testosterone on libido, mood and cognitive or memory performance (www.jeanhailes.org.au/research/current).

As the demand for HRT falls, it is expected that the drug companies will be searching for a new 'miracle' drug to capture this lost market. As I mentioned in the previous chapter, the female version of Viagra is one possible new 'miracle' drug. Other possibilities include antidepressants and testosterone (see p. 38). There is significant interest internationally in the area of testosterone research in women, and presently Australia leads the world in this field. Studies are currently underway at the Jean Hailes Foundation to determine how testosterone influences mood, libido and cognitive function in postmenopausal women, and the role of testosterone therapy for premenopausal women (Davis, 2003).

Although no form of testosterone therapy is currently approved for use in women in Australia by the Therapeutic Goods Administration, testosterone therapy has been used in Australia for women with low testosterone levels for many years. Information for GPs and health professionals on the Jean Hailes website explains how testosterone therapy can be administered. It reads:

> Testosterone can be taken as tablets, by injection, as an implanted pellet, as a skin patch, gel or spray. The most commonly used form of therapy for women has been with a

testosterone implant pellet. This is a very small pellet which is implanted in the fat of the front lower abdomen, using a small incision (less than 1 cm). The procedure takes approximately ten minutes to perform. The pellet releases testosterone over a period of 3 to 6 months, after which time it needs to be replaced. We most commonly recommend the use of 50 mg of the testosterone implant, although rarely 100 mg is required (www.jeanhailes.org.au/health_prof/hp_test_for_women.htm).

Despite the fact that testosterone is yet to receive approval for use in women in Australia, research studies are being conducted at what appears to be an incredible pace. It seems the race for a new miracle drug has begun. If a drug can be found that has wide appeal, then pharmaceutical companies will be recouping the losses from HRT. Let's hope that we have all learnt valuable lessons from the Women's Health Initiative.

Since the promise of a 'youth pill' through which, according to Robert Wilson, menopause could be avoided and ageing alleviated, women have turned towards HRT in search of the promise of eternal youth. Coney claims that it is the preoccupation with the restoration of youth, beauty and [hetero]sexual prowess that is responsible for the success of the HRT-awareness campaign (1993). As women in the Westernised world can now expect to live at least one third of their life after menopause, they make up a large market of potential HRT consumers. Pharmaceutical companies therefore stand to gain massive financial benefits as a consequence of the ageing female population (Berger, 1999).

A French study found that the amount of attention women pay to beauty care plays a role in determining HRT use. This study was a prospective survey, which consisted of three separate questionnaires in 1990, 1993 and 1996 (Fauconnier et al., 2000, 216). The study began in 1990 with 1262 women, and the follow-up cohort consisted of 940 women who responded to the 1993 and 1996 questionnaires. Six questions in the 1996 questionnaire explored representations of menopause, six questions explored beauty care practices and five questions from the 1990 survey explored women's expectations of HRT use. As usual, sexual orientation was not noted and hetero-sexuality was again assumed.

Results showed '. . . a positive linear relationship between the level of beauty care and HRT use, independent of other factors associated with HRT use' (Fauconnier et al., 2000, 224). While the authors acknowledge that the small difference in users and non-users of HRT and beauty care practices may not represent an important difference in behaviour, they nonetheless suggest '. . . the relationship between beauty care and HRT use should be compared with that which is observed between HRT use and expectations of anti-aging effects'. This study suggests that some women are using HRT as a cosmetic agent to counteract the physical signs of ageing. The authors point out that the cosmetic benefits of HRT are real, but this effect is minor and physicians should not consider it in determining whether HRT should be prescribed. From numerous responses received to my questionnaire, it appears that beauty care practices are not as important to many lesbians in my study as they are to many heterosexual women.

Conclusion

In this chapter I have discussed how the construction of menopause as a 'disease' has created a market for HRT as the 'cure'. Reasons women 'choose' or reject HRT are many and varied. The benefits and risks of HRT are confusing and conflicting. Women are undoubtedly confused about the value and risks of HRT and are often persuaded to commence HRT as a result of the media portrayal of its benefits and pressure placed on them by the medical profession. Women are often made to feel that taking HRT is the responsible course of action in regard to managing their menopause and life thereafter.

Without doubt, the release of the findings from the WHI in July 2002 has had a significant impact on the number of women taking and ceasing HRT. This is not, however, the end of the HRT story. The many contradictions, including the ways in which the media report them, make it extremely difficult for women to decide whether to take HRT for short-term use or to try other remedies should their menopausal 'symptoms' make life difficult.

Importantly, studies which have explored women's views and experiences of HRT have failed to acknowledge sexual orientation as a variable, and have assumed heterosexuality. In contrast, the women in my research explore the views, experiences and attitudes towards HRT from lesbians' perspectives.

5

Health services and homophobia

In this chapter, I discuss lesbians' experiences with the health system and other issues related to lesbian health research and practice, and I critically examine the Australian and international literature on this topic. Although there is a growing amount of lesbian research emerging from Australia, the majority of research in this area has been conducted in the US. Research in the past has focused on the views of health professionals and the health-seeking behaviours of lesbians, but very few studies have looked at the issues from the lesbians' own perspectives. In this chapter I will present the voices of the participants in my study and reflect on their experiences with – and views of – the mainstream health system in Australia during the first years of the twenty-first century.

The vast majority of lesbian-related research has been conducted by lesbians and for this very reason it is often viewed as invalid or biased. It is interesting how this 'insider' perspective is used to discredit the work conducted by lesbians. When research has been conducted on men by white male researchers, this work is seldom seen as invalid or biased. On the contrary, this 'insider status' is said to strengthen the research and shows authority. Often, issues that are seen to be 'marginal' are given more credibility when pursued by members of the dominant or powerful group. In the case of lesbian health, the dominant/powerful group is the heterosexual population. Unfortunately for lesbian health, heterosexuals are not always interested in this topic. My own professional experience provides evidence to support this claim. While working at a regional women's health service, I attempted to raise the profile of lesbian health issues. The health service did not provide any specific programs for lesbians, which was in my view a blatant omission. The service did, however, provide a range of innovative health programs for women with disabilities and women from culturally and linguistically diverse backgrounds. Lesbians, like members of any minority group, are often seen to be 'pushing their own barrow' when pursuing areas of interest and relevance to members of their group. Frequently I was asked why I was concerned with lesbian health issues and why I saw the necessity to highlight my own needs and concerns at my workplace. As a white, educated, middle-class lesbian I am fortunate to have options, choices and resources available to me that are denied to many other lesbians. It is important, I believe, that those of us who have the necessary resources (human, financial, other) work to ensure that the women's voices that would not otherwise be heard are in fact made public. For these reasons I think it is crucial that lesbian health is firmly placed on the women's health agenda. Usually it is lesbians who see this need and make it part of the women's health business. This analysis, however, was often lost on many of my heterosexual colleagues, although I am happy to report that the service now provides programs and events that are targeted to lesbians. I find it disappointing, however, that these changes in service direction came about only after I left the organisation and heterosexual women were driving the lesbian health agenda.

At the time of writing this book, very few health services are providing lesbian-specific services and programs in the state of Victoria, and in Australia in general, particularly in rural areas.

When such programs are provided, their focus is invariably aimed at younger lesbians. Older lesbians remain invisible within both mainstream and women's health services.

Findings from my study confirm those of larger studies and support the view that homophobia is widespread throughout mainstream health services.

Homophobia is defined as the 'irrational fear of, aversion to, or discrimination against homosexuality or homosexuals' (Merriam-Webster, 1993, 556). Heterosexism is the belief that heterosexuality is the only acceptable form of sexuality. Homophobic attitudes appear to be widespread throughout the entire health system, and are not related to one occupational group, although in my study participants frequently singled out medical practitioners. There are many different examples of how homophobia is played out within the health system. In the following pages, I discuss some of these examples.

In the year 2000, the Royal Women's Hospital in Victoria, Australia, undertook a Lesbian Health Information Project (LHIP) in an attempt to assess the literature and health experiences of lesbians. It was hoped that the findings of this project would inform future hospital directions, and improve and expand the existing services to ensure access for lesbians. The hospital's health promotion program, *absolutely women's health*, has maintained a focus on lesbian health and wellbeing and regularly hosts forums and events that are relevant to the needs and interests of many lesbians in the general community (see www.rwh.org.au/wellwomens/awh.cfm). This is a unique and innovative women's health promotion program located within a large tertiary public hospital.

The Lesbian Health Information Project (LHIP) collected data from interviews, focus groups and questionnaires between April and July 2000. Interviews and focus groups were conducted with 120 lesbian consumers, 80 hospital staff and 25 external health professionals. According to the data obtained, lesbians commonly reported experiencing homophobia and heterosexism, combined with the assumption of hetero-sexuality, when accessing health care. Lesbians were concerned about the lack of knowledge regarding lesbian health issues and the lack of sensitivity displayed by health service providers (Brown, 2000).

Lesbians' dissatisfaction with the health system

A review of the international literature on lesbian health care reveals interesting and disturbing findings. US nurse researchers Patricia Stevens and Joanne Hall assert that in order to provide quality nursing care to lesbians, it is important that nurses have an understanding of the cultural context of lesbian lives and a knowledge of what illness and wellness means for lesbians. It is also important that nurses and other health care professionals have some understanding of the issues lesbians frequently experience when accessing health care. My own research has shown that many health professionals do not possess this level of knowledge and understanding.

Stevens and Hall conducted a study to investigate the concepts of health and illness among lesbians. Twenty-five self-identified lesbians were recruited through a snowballing tech-nique from the lesbian community in Iowa. The participants were white, college-educated, employed, and aged from 21 to 58 years. The authors acknowledge the potentially biased sample in that the majority of the women were assertive and open and accepting of their lesbian identity.

Semi-structured interviews were conducted with the participants focussing on lesbians' identifiability, health strengths and weaknesses, and interactions with health care providers. Findings revealed that 48 per cent of participants believed they were clearly identifiable to everyone as lesbians, while 20 per cent believed that no one could tell. The authors point out that as some of the participants believe that their lesbianism is obvious to others, these women develop ways to minimise the negative impact of the stigma. Stevens and Hall write:

> The means by which a lesbian believes her identity to be revealed may affect how she values such aspects of herself as body image, associations and personality characteristics. Her attitude toward the degree of identifiability she attributes to herself may be related to the degree of self-affirmation that she has as a lesbian. Her sense of control over the disclosure of her lesbian identity may be related to the level of stress that she experiences. For example, both the woman who believes that she can conceal her lesbian identity and the woman who behaves as though she is highly identifiable may experience a sense of control and thereby reduce stress (1988, 71).

Participants in this study viewed health as a holistic concept and regarded independence and self-reliance as key determinants of wellness. Women spoke of their distress about ageing and regarded it as a time of loss of physical, economic and social independence – all of which were central to their definition of wellness. Most participants worried about becoming dependant on others as they aged and many anticipated alienation due to a lack of social support services for older lesbians. Interestingly, many feared an increased reliance on the mainstream health system because of a mistrust of the safety and appropriateness of its ability to care for lesbians. The participants in this study did not address the issue of menopause.

Participants' responses to questions about communication with health care providers also related to stigmatised identity. Seventy-two per cent of respondents described negative responses from their provider once their sexual orientation was known. These responses included shock, embarrassment, fear, pity, invasive personal questioning, unfriendliness, rough physical handling, partners being mistreated and breaches of confidentiality. Thirty-six per cent of the respondents mentioned instances where they terminated the discussion and/or refused to return to that particular provider due to responses received after disclosure. The following quote illustrates the point well:

> As soon as I said I was a lesbian, the nurses started giving me disgusted looks. They were nasty to my partner. They rough-housed me. They were not gentle like they would be to a straight woman. They treated me like I was 'one of those,' like they might catch something (Stevens and Hall, 1988, 72).

These responses are similar to those I received in answer to my questions about lesbians' experiences with the health system. The topics of homophobia and lesbians' experiences of the health system were crucial to my study. Questionnaire and interview responses revealed that over half of the lesbians in my research project (52.6 per cent) had experienced homophobia when interacting with the health system. Many lesbians in my study wrote and spoke freely about negative experiences with the health system and several offered strategies for improvement. This information came from both the questionnaire and interview data. Few of the lesbians who experienced homophobia at the hands of health professionals felt able to challenge these behaviours and instead chose not to return to that particular health professional. Of all sections on the questionnaire, health services and homophobia received the most additional comments. Some examples of homophobia reported on the questionnaire data include:

> Once during an internal examination I jumped when the male doctor literally stuck the speculum into me – his sneering voice said, 'most women like it'. Even the nurse was shocked! [125]

> In A&E [Accident and Emergency] after an accident, the nurse presumed my straight girlfriend and I were lovers. She treated the scrubbing of my deeply grazed back overzealously until my friend left the room to phone her husband! The nurse was

apologetic UNTIL I explained that only my friend was hetero and not me! [118]

Recently, I accompanied my partner to the local emergency department for treatment of an acute asthma attack. The triage nurse, seeing the difficulty my partner was having breathing, took us straight into the resuscitation area. When the nurse asked for my partner's details and I indicated I was her partner and next of kin, her attitude changed dramatically. I could barely believe the change in her attitude. She had been so kind and caring and now she was hostile, rude and rough. My partner is employed at this hospital and she pleaded with me not to make a formal complaint. [27]

Other comments, which may seem not as extreme, none-theless, clearly demonstrate homophobic views and attitudes. These include:

When I asked about safe sex practices for lesbians I was given a list of venereal diseases. [48]

One GP I went to (I think for Pap Smear) said how much he preferred treating lesbians as we were so 'clean', meaning I presume, that we were unsullied by penis penetration or sperm. I never went back to him. [156]

Just as Patricia Stevens and Joanne Hall found in their study, I also found an overwhelming assumption of heterosexuality; participants in my study also remarked on this issue. Health professionals and questions on standard medical forms continue to assume a heterosexual orientation. Questions relating to marital status, contraception used and [hetero]-sexual activity, all highlight the heterosexist bias inherent in the health system. The following quote from the questionnaire data illustrates this point well:

I had an STD from a female partner and the doctor asked me to give this medication to my male partner. I said to the doctor

I don't have a male partner. I have this problem from a woman and he looked at me with utter complete disgust and said to me, 'I would like you to leave my surgery and I'd prefer it if you found another doctor to treat you, don't come back to this clinic again'. [179]

Other participants provided ideas as to how to change the heterosexist bias within the health services and many offered practical strategies to do this. For example:

Look at the language on health leaflets, etc. Remove all references to husband/wife. Look at images of couples; some could be same sex. Forms for completion should be reviewed to ensure questions, options and language used is inclusive. Doctors and other health professionals training should include how to ask open or inclusive questions rather than hetero-sexually based. [25]

Policy needs to be inclusive in its language. Practitioners need to be offered awareness training. More lesbian focussed resources. [6]

Many lesbians in my study shared similar views on this topic. From the responses received, the majority of lesbians who wrote and spoke about this issue felt strongly that health professionals need to be more aware of language they use when interacting with women, as is evidenced in Alison's remarks:

From my experience with the medical system, all women are generally viewed as straight by doctors unless you out yourself to them. It would be better if the issue of partners was a first line, routine question for GPs as this would set a more accepting parameter for the usual following routine questions. I feel as if I need to be on guard when I see a health practitioner to out myself or wait for an assumption to be made and then I have to correct it. I also feel that often I have to look after the GP if her/his reaction is one of shock. Unfortunately we have a limited choice of health practitioners available here in the country.

Participants in Stevens and Hall's study expressed the view that there was '. . . no routine, comfortable way to let health care providers know that heterosexual assumptions were not applicable to them as lesbians' (1988, 72). In order to avoid being represented as heterosexual when they were not, many participants felt they were forced to come out to their provider. Ninety-six per cent of participants mentioned situations where it could be harmful to them if the provider knew of their lesbian identity. Lesbians spoke of having to assess each individual encounter with health care providers and having to make an assessment as to whether to disclose or not. Not surprisingly, given these experiences, 84 per cent of the study participants stated that they were reluctant to seek out health care. This figure has been supported in other studies from the US, New Zealand and, more recently, Australia. This reluctance to seek care raises serious concerns about access of health care services to lesbians and I believe needs to be urgently addressed. According to Stevens and Hall, the participants believe that:

. . . dispelling heterosexual assumption and eliminating prejudicial attitude and action is the responsibility of health care providers so that health care can be made accessible to lesbians. With empathy and accurate information about lesbians, participants felt it would be possible for health care providers to overcome their negative responses. However, they wanted providers to have dealt with the issue before that moment when it comes to providing care to them (1988, 73).

Participants in my study spoke of the reluctance to seek out medical care due to the homophobic attitudes of many health professionals. As previously stated, over half the participants reported experiencing homophobia and/or heterosexism in their interactions with health professionals. It must be noted that of the 47.4 per cent who had not experienced such interactions, almost 30 per cent of these women were not out to their health providers.

Not being out, however, does not ensure a discrimination- and homophobic-free consultation. If a lesbian is not out about her sexuality, she will be assumed to be heterosexual and will therefore remain invisible as a lesbian within the health system (McNair & Dyson, 1999). Seventy-one per cent of lesbians in my sample believe that lesbians are invisible within the Westernised medical model, whilst 40.5 per cent suggest that lesbians are invisible within the 'alternative/complementary' health system. The issue of invisibility was one of the most commonly mentioned themes throughout my study. Many lesbians spoke of the need to discuss relationship/sexual issues with medical practitioners yet felt that because of fear of discrimination it was not safe for them to do so. The following questionnaire responses highlight these concerns:

> The doctor never asked me how menopause was affecting my sexual relationship but I bet she would've asked a married heterosexual woman. [69]

And another woman wrote:

> Doctors are willing to discuss sexual issues relating to meno-pause if you have a husband but if you don't have a husband you can't have a sex life so there's nothing to discuss. [136]

An opposing viewpoint suggests that lesbians' invisibility within the health service is due to a lesbian's lack of openness and honesty with her health provider. While this view may be interpreted as 'blaming the victim', some lesbians I inter-viewed believed strongly that if change is to occur, then it will only come from lesbians as consumers, not from health professionals. Elizabeth told me:

We make ourselves invisible, I think. Like, there are plenty of women's clinics and gay- and lesbian-friendly clinics, for example and there are opportunities for people to receive good medical care either through their local clinics or through specialist clinics. I just . . . you would hope that they would recall your case history and realise that you're a lesbian and not talk to you about birth control during this time. So, as a lesbian, I guess if you want to receive good medical treatment you need to be out in a sense that you need to have explained your situation to the doctor, because I think if you hadn't and the doctor asked about birth control, because this is a time when you can be falling pregnant, and you got really upset about that because you're not having sex with a male, then to a certain extent it is your own fault for not explaining to the doctor that you're in fact a lesbian. It's like that we're a patriarchal society even though we're working hard all the time. Like, I just feel that I have a responsibility to educate . . . as a confident lesbian I have a responsibility to educate.

Elizabeth is a well-educated, assertive, professional woman who has a background in nursing. She acknowledges that she is confident and realises that this impacts on the level and extent of communication she has with her health providers. She further explained:

I've been to a gynaecologist and he said, 'What are you using for birth control?' and I said, 'I'm not using anything; I'm a lesbian,' and he just didn't blink. It was no big deal. He obviously treats lots of lesbians. *** is a major town.[1] It has a population of 20 000. He'd come across lots of people from lots of diverse backgrounds, so there's no problem and I don't get asked those questions from either my GP or a specialist. So there's no issue there for me, but I'm confident too.

Jill shared Elizabeth's views and spoke of the roles assertiveness and self-knowledge play in getting what is needed in terms of good health care. Jill wrote on the questionnaire:

Assertiveness is an absolute prerequisite to getting health advice/care; so is self-knowledge about our own bodies/health. Otherwise we can be so badly advised/diagnosed/treated we can die. As an ex-nurse, that is, someone with an 'insider' view of the health system, I am appalled by the Western medical approach to our health overall and avoid it like the plague. [58]

Similarly, another participant wrote:

By stating my sexuality at the outset everyone is aware of my individual needs and no assumptions are made. Being out with medical practitioners and services, I believe, improves awareness and improves service delivery. [176]

However, some lesbians in my study did not regard disclosure of their sexual identity to their health provider an option. This appeared to be particularly so for lesbians living in rural and remote communities. The following quote from the questionnaire data illustrate this point:

Every local medical service I have had dealings with assumes I am heterosexual and married. They call me 'Mrs' despite being told several times 'Ms'. I cannot trust a positive reaction to my disclosure of my sexuality so I choose not to in this town. [35]

I prefer not to out myself unless I am sure that I will be accepted and treated with respect. [129]

A nurse who lives in a small town and is not out to her primary health provider, explained, 'It is a very small town and the receptionist has a big mouth.' [167]

I asked participants to rate their overall experiences of the health system and gave them the categories of 'good', 'fair', 'poor', 'excellent', 'average', 'less than satisfactory', or 'other'.[2] Less than half of the participants indicated that their experiences had been 'good' (45 per cent), almost one quarter replied 'average' (22.4 per cent), 'fair' (9 per cent), excellent (8 per cent), and four per cent indicated 'poor'. Five per cent of lesbians in this sample stated that their experiences had been 'less than satisfactory' and six per cent ticked 'other'.

I gave women the option of writing additional comments about their experiences with the health system on the questionnaire and many took up this option. These comments and personal anecdotes were mixed in terms of positive and negative remarks. A registered nurse who indicated that her experiences with the health system had been 'poor', wrote:

Despite above [poor experiences] there have been some wonderful health professionals who have challenged their internalised homophobia since I have known them and with whom I have experienced healthy professional relationships – not all women I must say. [1]

Another participant explains:

My experiences have been less than satisfactory – incomplete or unhelpful assessments, sometimes due to poor understanding about lesbians and what is important. In other instances I haven't been given all information because I didn't say anything about being a lesbian. Sometimes it has been all of the thinking style that is attached to Western medicine. [72]

This woman went on to explain how shocked and surprised she was when a doctor asked her a question about her sexual orientation. She writes:

I was shocked once when a doctor asked me if I had ever been heterosexual! I later found she was a lesbian but this is the *only example* [her emphasis] in all my experience when such a question was included at an initial consultation. [72]

A woman who indicated that her experiences with the health system had been 'downright disgusting' wrote:

Misdiagnosed and under-serviced due to being fat. Fobbed off as a depressed neurotic for being assertive and not accepting their word as law. Fat, female, lesbian and over fifty all affect my experiences. I have a lot of anger about how I have been treated over the years. I'm still sorting through it all. [43]

Another woman remarked:

Generally I'm a confident, assertive, informed user of health systems and been well responded to across several interactions with Western medicine. If my lesbian identity has been known, it has not, in my eyes, impinged on how I've been treated. My experience has generally been good but I've had good control over how I interact with it, never having been seriously ill or reliant on health providers for big stuff. I'm not as sure about safety as a lesbian if I were seriously ill. [5]

Kate lives in a rural community where there is a shortage of general practitioners generally and a shortage of female GPs in particular. In an interview Kate explained to me how the medical practice she visits has 'closed its books' to new patients and will only see people who reside in the immediate area. Kate told me how her friend who lives in a nearby town wanted to see the local female doctor but did not have a local address. Kate explains:

A woman that I recently met who is straight and lives down the road wanted to come up to that surgery because she wanted a female doctor. All the female doctors in *** had closed their books because they all work part-time, but you had to have a local address. I said she could use mine, and anyway, she got in. I saw her and she goes, 'Oh, I saw this doctor,' and I go, 'Yeah, I heard she's really good.' 'Oh, she actually asked me a very strange question.' The two of us were just sitting there and we go, 'Why?' She said, 'Oh, she asked me was I heterosexual or homosexual. Why would she ask me that?' And we went, 'That's fantastic,' and she just didn't get it. She was really offended. So the other woman that was with me was straight, and her and I both went on about why she would've asked that. We talked about lesbian health and Pap smears and breast-screening and blah blah and she had no awareness whatsoever what it was like for lesbians. So it was brilliant! [44]

Such open-minded health professionals unfortunately appear to be the exception rather than the rule. This female doctor was a locum filling in for a short time from the city. Attitudes and questions such as these asked by doctors will contribute towards eliminating homophobia and may lead to a better quality of health service for all.

Although I acknowledge that this self-rating experience is highly subjective, the findings nevertheless indicate a general dissatisfaction with the mainstream or medical model of healthcare. These results have significant implications for health providers and health services generally.

Lesbians' health-seeking behaviour

Many studies have focused on the health-seeking behaviour of lesbians. US researchers Jocelyn White and Valerie Dull designed a study to investigate lesbians' health risk factors and their health-seeking behaviours. Respondents were recruited from a convenience sample of women attending a lesbian health conference in Oregon, US and the readership of a lesbian community newsletter. A total of 324 women responded to a four-part questionnaire. The women self-identified as lesbians (287), bisexual (15) and 'no identity' or 'other' (10).[3] The first part of the questionnaire related to specific health issues such as cancers, substance abuse, weight, nutrition, coming out, violence, menopause, suicide, HIV, heart disease and others. The second part asked questions related to the ease or difficulty in obtaining health care and health-seeking behaviours. The third section focused on the women's levels of comfort or discomfort when discussing sensitive issues with their health care provider. The final section related to demographic information and provided space for additional comments.

The mean age of the lesbians in the sample was 41 years and 84.6 per cent of the lesbians were Caucasian. Participants were well educated, with over 58 per cent of respondents having more than a college-level education. The majority of the women were employed in full-time paid employment and 89.5 per cent had health insurance. The authors acknowledge this bias in their sample and accept that this group may not be typical of lesbians in the general population. The respondents belonged to a community organisation that incorporated lesbian health into its mission statement, consequently the women's health-related behaviours might differ from that of lesbians in the general community.

The study found that the fewer male partners a lesbian had during her lifetime, the greater appeared her health risk. While this appears to be a surprising finding, the authors suggest the reason for this is that heterosexual women, who are sexually active with men, regularly attend medical consultations for issues such as birth control and Pap tests and thus frequently receive health checks and other preventative health measures. The authors suggest that lesbians who are exclusively having sex with women might be missing out on regular women's health screening. A possible explanation, according to researchers, is that these women do not present at primary care clinics as frequently as heterosexual women who may have a need for birth control. This raises concerns about lesbians' knowledge of the need for screening services and access to appropriate health care providers and, according to the authors, has negative effects on their general health. It must be pointed out that as medical researchers, Jocelyn White and Valerie Dull reflect a medicalised view of health screening and prevention. An alternative view would suggest that the fewer male partners a woman has during her lifetime, the lower would be the risk of sexually transmitted infections (STIs) and the less likely she is to suffer from the damaging effects of many types of contraceptives. Lesbian sexual health research has consistently found lower rates of STIs among women who have sex exclusively with women than compared with their heterosexually active counterparts. It must be pointed out, however, that although the risk of STIs is lower between women, it is still possible to transmit certain infections between women, and thus, 'low risk' is not the same as 'no risk' (Wilton, 2000).

Findings from Jocelyn White and Valerie Dull's study suggest that a proportion of lesbians are relying on their partner for health information and they may be replacing advice from doctors and other health care professionals with advice from their partners. White and Dull acknowledge that partners offer a great deal of support to each other, but argue that they must not replace the care and information provided by health professionals. They suggest that lesbians need to be encouraged to take their partners to their health care provider and they should be involved in the care. However, as other studies have reported, when lesbians have followed this suggestion, they often experience negative treatment.

These research findings support those of previous studies that confirm that the interaction between the client and her provider is a major determinant in health-seeking behaviour of lesbians. Lesbians are more likely to seek health care if they perceive the health care provider to be sensitive and competent. Many of my research participants supported this finding. One of the participants in my study summed this point up well when she wrote on the questionnaire:

I want to go to a health professional where I am not educating them, where I am treated and respected as me. [59]

More than half of the participants in my study reported that their health provider identifies as gay- and lesbian-friendly

(59.4 per cent). Many lesbians living in cities commented how they prefer to use the services of a known gay- and lesbian-friendly health provider. These services, however, are not commonly found outside major cities. Lesbians who live in rural and remote locations rarely have this option. In many smaller communities the option of a female doctor is often not a possibility, let alone a gay- and lesbian-friendly one.

Not surprisingly, a large number of lesbians in this study were travelling vast distances to see the doctor of their choice. In a focus group I conducted in 2001 with lesbians from a rural area in the state of Victoria, 12 out of the 14 participants stated that they travel out of their immediate local area regularly to visit a general practitioner (GP).[4] The lesbians remarked that they had been dissatisfied with their interaction with the nearest GP and thus preferred to travel to find a doctor they felt comfortable with. One woman travels more than 80 kilometres to the city to visit her gay- and lesbian-friendly GP.

Of the 92 lesbians in my study who have a regular GP, 51 per cent indicated they travel a distance to see their preferred doctor rather than consulting the nearest doctor available. Distances women travelled ranged from five kilometres to 950 kilometres. Responses from the questionnaire data include:

If possible I travel from Brisbane to Sydney [approximately 950 kilometres/590 miles] to see my GP although that is not always possible. [125]

I travel from *** to Melbourne [a distance of approximately 100 kilometres/62 miles] as the local GPs seem narrow, suburban and limited. [21]

And another woman wrote:

She was my local doctor and I have kept seeing her when I moved away. I now live 150 kilometres away and I will be moving to a local doctor soon. The problem is that the local

132

lesbian doctor's books are closed and that is why I keep going back to my old doctor. [34]

Not all respondents indicated the distances travelled to see their preferred doctor although most gave reasons for their choices. Some of the reasons stated include:

I travel because she is comfortable with my sexuality and the choices I have made such as having a child via self-insemination. She is also very competent in the clinical stuff as well as an excellent communicator. I have worked hard to find practitioners I feel will accept my lesbianism. We pay the price by having to be ever-vigilant. As a lesbian and a single mother it is very hard to find bulk-billing GPs in our community and alternative health is very expensive. [172]

I travel 10 kilometres because she is a lesbian. [3]

My GP is a lesbian and the distance is 15 kilometres from home. [1]

Up to 10 kilometres because it is gay- and lesbian-friendly and there is a sense of community. [45]

Thirty kilometres for suitable female doctor who is lesbian-friendly and understanding of my history and medical conditions. [30]

30 minutes because recommended as gay-friendly and female-focussed and good care. Also is a naturopath. [60]

Another US study compared the health risk behaviour, health status and access and barriers to health care among lesbians, bisexual and heterosexual women. Allison Diamant and her colleagues used a public access data file compiled from the Los Angeles County Health Survey. The research sample consisted of 4697 women, of whom 51 self-identified as lesbian, 36 as bisexual and 4610 as heterosexual. The mean age of women in this sample was 42 years. The authors acknowledge the small number of lesbians in their sample, however, they cite a statistic that claims lesbians comprise 1.0 – 3.6 per cent[5] of the US female population and assert that if this finding is accurate, then their sample size of 51 lesbians and 36 bisexual women may in fact be representative of Los Angeles County's population.

Findings revealed that there were significant differences in the receipt of preventative health care services and that lesbians and bisexual women experience greater barriers to accessing medical care than their heterosexual counterparts. Lesbians and bisexual women were less likely to have health insurance and this was a definite barrier to accessing medical care. Similarly, lesbians and bisexual women were less likely to have a private physician as their regular health provider. The authors argue that this may be related to the low numbers of lesbians and bisexual women with health insurance.

Audrey Koh, a US obstetrician/gynaecologist, designed a study to determine whether lesbians and bisexual women are less likely than heterosexual women to use preventative health measures (Koh, 2000). This study, the first to compare the health of lesbian, bisexual and heterosexual women in the same setting, and the first large study to describe the experiences of lesbian, bisexual and heterosexual women who use the healthcare system, provided interesting results. Participants included 524 lesbians, 123 bisexual women and 637 heterosexual women. The settings were in 33 physicians' offices and community health clinics in urban areas of 13 states across the US. The results showed that lesbians and bisexual women were less likely to use preventative health measures than heterosexual women. The author suggests lesbians and bisexual women use the health care system less than heterosexual women because they may have lower rates of income and lower rates of health insurance. However, as other research studies have identified, they are also less likely to need antenatal and contraceptive care. Importantly, many of these women avoid contact with the system, as they fear discrimination due to their sexual orientation. Koh points out that other studies have shown that lesbians are likely to use complementary healthcare providers if they are seeking holistic and less-discriminatory care.[6]

In my own study I was interested in lesbians' health-seeking behaviour and I included several questions to gather some Australian data on this topic. Questionnaire responses reveal that women in my study were relying on a variety of health providers and diverse sources for information related to menopause. Seventy-seven per cent of lesbians in this study had consulted a health professional about their menopause, while 21.5 per cent had not.

Lesbians in my study were asked to nominate the type of health care provider they regard as their primary provider and their responses listed a wide range of health providers. As other studies have reported, lesbians are likely to use a range of health providers in their search for more holistic and less discriminatory care. Almost one quarter of participants in my study (24 per cent) rely on a combination of health care providers rather than one primary care provider. Some of these health providers include: general practitioners (GPs), naturopaths, Chinese herbalists, acupuncturists, nurses, homoeopaths, masseurs, chiropractors and staff at menopause clinics. Other ways in which lesbians in this study sought information about menopause-related issues were by means of talking circles at lesbian gatherings and conferences, women's health centres, partners, friends, their mothers, books, websites, ABC radio, Radio National, lesbian and general women's magazines, and journals.

Seventy-nine per cent of lesbians in my study have a regular general practitioner (GP). Sixty per cent of participants nominated a GP as their primary health provider. Naturopaths were identified as the primary health provider by six per cent of lesbians in the sample and four per cent nominated a chiropractor as their primary provider. Five per cent of respondents stated 'other' as their primary provider and did not define the type of provider. Lesbians were asked their reasons for using a range of 'alternative' providers and responses mirrored those of other studies. From the questionnaire data, it appears that many lesbians in this study view the medical model as narrow and 'symptom-orientated', rather than reflecting a holistic approach. For example, study participants wrote:

I think that Western medicine treats the result not the cause. It treats ageing as death, as enemy, not natural progressions and it is very out of touch with the human state and interferes too much. I try to stay away. [3]

Alternative medicine works on the causes whereas Western medicine works to alleviate the symptoms regardless of what other body damage occurs. [43]

A major problem with traditional Western medicine is compartmentalisation, i.e will only look at one bit of the body at a time (the offending bit) – doesn't look for relationships between bits. [190]

Western medicine has a good place for acute needs. For whole body considerations we need access to broader understandings. Our bodies are complex and limited outlooks are not helpful. [72]

Western medicine is good for accidents, setting broken bones and diagnosis, not much else. [16]

Sometimes doctors have too narrow a view of the body – I don't agree that the medical model is the only one that works. [130]

Other women explained how they consult different health providers for different health conditions and related issues. For example:

I tend to seek different health providers for different health problems. I choose naturopathy first but sometimes I need a doctor or chiropractor. [128]

Acupuncturist is best for tissue injuries, naturopath and homoeopath best for hormone balance and general metabolism. The GP is for Pap smears, blood tests, vaccinations and medical certificates. [133]

I have over my life used natural therapy but usually when I see someone it's for a medical certificate rather than treatment. [148]

Homoeopathy is the most effective modality for me. I also use a GP for prescriptions and standard health information. [187]

Acupuncture is wonderful, I believe in its fundamentals of energy flows, and energy blocks, which result in ill being. My GP is for quick-fix issues, i.e. infection, aches and pains. [27]

Some women mentioned the mind/body/spiritual balance and indicated they use a range of providers and treatments in an attempt to regain balance and alignment. One woman wrote:

I believe that when things are not working properly (illness or disease) then I need to realign my bodies (spiritual, mental, emotional, physical) with natural remedies and lots of rest/sleep, meditation and being in nature. [68]

And similarly:

Doctor is for prescriptions and monitoring of my osteoporosis; naturopath is my 'witch-sister' who discusses more spiritual aspects of healing and gives me rescue remedy. [197]

One woman commented:

Allopathic medicine seems to me to be fundamentally corrupted by the investments in profit (pharmaceutical companies and multinationals). [38]

Nathalia was explicit in her judgment:

Mainstream medicine is fucked and only good for emergencies.

These questionnaire responses illustrate a general dissatis-faction with the medical model. Mostly, medical practitioners are sought out for 'quick fix' approaches and/or compulsory medical certificates, while alternative practitioners are consulted for realigning mind and body.

I was interested to learn about lesbians' preventative health behaviours. As other studies have demonstrated, lesbians are less likely than heterosexual women to seek routine preven-tative health care. Questions relating to preventative health behaviours in this study were restricted to Pap tests and BreastScreen. Results from my questionnaire provide new information about an Australian sample of lesbians and their health-seeking behaviours. Fifty-eight women (50 per cent of total participants) in this study were fifty years of age and over at the time of completing the questionnaire and therefore eligible to attend the National Program for the Early Detection of Breast Cancer (BreastScreen). Out of an eligible population for BreastScreen, almost one-third of lesbians were not accessing this service. These results are similar to those published in larger, international studies. As lesbians are considered to be at a possible higher risk for breast cancer, this finding may have significant implications (see p. 157).

In relation to cervical cancer, studies have shown that the interval between Pap tests is nearly three times longer for lesbians than for heterosexual women (Gruskin, 1999; O'Hanlan, 1995). A Melbourne-based study designed to assess lesbians' cervical screening history and experiences found that sixty-six per cent of respondents were well screened, twenty-two per cent were under-screened and twelve per cent had never had a Pap test (Brown et al., 2002). These results came from a self-report survey that was completed at a large annual gay and lesbian community event. Findings from my study differ in terms of the percentage of lesbians who have never had a Pap test. Over 70 per cent of lesbians in my study reported having two-yearly Pap tests, whilst 29.3 per cent reported not having Pap tests at all. This inconsistency with the international data may reflect the higher educational level and/or the fact that many women in my sample are employed in the health care industry (75.4 per cent tertiary educated and 39.4 per cent health workers).[7]

Health practitioners' knowledge and attitude towards lesbian health

Patricia Stevens provides an overview of the existing research from 1970 to 1990 about health care professionals' attitudes towards lesbians as well as lesbians' experiences of the health care system (Stevens, 1992). Stevens reviewed 19 published studies, which identify health provider bias and ignorance as common themes throughout. Lesbians commonly report health professionals to be rejecting, hostile and abusive.

In Australia, Ruth McNair and Sue Dyson (1999) conducted a study in the state of Victoria to collect information about the general attitudes and knowledge among primary health providers in terms of lesbian health. Fifty-one practitioners participated in their study; the majority of whom were general practitioners (GPs),[8] however, a small number of allied health professionals[9] also participated. McNair and Dyson conducted six focus groups over several geographic areas in Victoria in order to involve a wide range of practitioners. They developed a series of questions which served as discussion points within the focus groups. Participants in the groups were male and female and their ages ranged from 20 to 62 years.

The focus group questions were divided into four distinct areas. These areas were:

- Assessing attitudes to lesbian patients and lesbian health;
- Knowledge of lesbian health issues;

- Strategies to increase awareness and knowledge;
- Overcoming barriers within primary health care to lesbians.

The authors report '. . . that the level of comfort in treating lesbian patients was refreshingly high' (1999, 3). Only two practitioners had not treated self-identified lesbians and others were aware that they saw lesbians who did not disclose their sexual orientation. Practitioners acknowledged a degree of discomfort when lesbians asked questions about a topic about which they had little knowledge. Some group participants spoke of witnessing examples of misogyny, yet very few had seen cases of obvious discrimination towards lesbian patients. Others had witnessed cases of discrimination towards gay male patients in the hospital setting, however, as McNair and Dyson point out, this in itself does not indicate a lack of homophobia; rather it suggests that lesbians remain invisible within the system.

Many studies conclude that it is important for the health practitioner to know the client/patient's sexual orientation in order to provide high quality and appropriate primary care. The exact percentage of women who are lesbians is difficult to determine. Surveys estimate that between 2 per cent and 10 per cent of the population are women who are sexually active with women. As it is impossible to know a woman's sexual orientation unless she discloses this information, it is important and indeed necessary for health care providers to use language that is free from heterosexual bias when working with women. Many participants in my study made this point strongly as is evident from the following sample of some of the questionnaire responses:

Never assume heterosexuality, as happened to me. [2]

Doctors and other health professionals' training should include how to ask open or inclusive questions rather than heterosexual-based. [25]

Provide more education to health professionals about our lifestyles and urge them to be more accepting of us. [1]

Do not assume we are straight. Recognise significant events in our lives that impact on our health. [9]

Every medical person must accept that gay isn't a disease. [19]

The issue of disclosure of sexual preference in McNair and Dyson's study gave interesting results. All focus group participants believed it was important to know the sexual preference of the patient in certain situations (particularly in relation to sexual problems, sexually transmitted diseases and gynaecological problems), yet none of the participants routinely asked their female patients. Two of the participants routinely asked male patients. McNair and Dyson conclude that there is reluctance on behalf of the practitioner to ask their female patients about their sexual preference. This reluctance, the authors suggest, is due to fear of offending heterosexual patients and, due to a lack of skill in asking in a sensitive and non-judgmental way. McNair and Dyson suggest that there is an expectation that lesbians will disclose their sexuality once they are comfortable with the provider, or if they believe it is relevant to the consultation. This, the authors claim, is in direct contrast to the approach taken by many of the lesbians who wait for signs that it is safe to come out to the provider before doing so. The result of this action is that only a third to half eventually disclose (1999, 4). Results from my study confirm this finding. One of my participants wrote on the questionnaire:

I prefer not to out myself unless I am sure that I will be accepted and treated with respect. [129]

McNair and Dyson term this the 'after you, no, after you' phenomenon, which they argue perpetuates lesbian invisibility within medical consultations. Focus group participants identified a range of issues they considered to be lesbian health issues. Menopause and other issues directly associated with older women were not identified. Health issues identified as lesbian health issues included Pap tests, mental health, fertility/parenting, STDs and safe sex, lesbian relationships, domestic violence, breast health, drug and alcohol use, sports injuries and access to services.

In my own study, I asked women about their reasons for not disclosing their sexual identity to their health providers and responses included: 'Fear of the response I may receive', 'I may then suffer discrimination', and 'I may not receive good care if she/he knows I am a lesbian', 'She/he will think differently of me', as well as 'It is not relevant'. These responses typify those of other larger international studies.

As a result of their study, McNair and Dyson suggest to practice positive discrimination, which, they believe, is preferable to self-disclosure. When I have asked services/organisations to consider including a new category on their medical and intake forms, so as to give women the option of disclosing their sexual orientation, and therefore indicating that the service acknowledges that not all women are heterosexual, I am frequently told that this inclusion might offend or alienate heterosexual women or that such information is simply irrelevant.

I argue that these comments reflect the service provider's heterosexism and homophobia. Such paternalistic views, I believe, are outdated and unhelpful. If women do not wish to out themselves on a form or in a consultation they simply will not do so. Presently, most standard intake forms do not present this as an option, and as a result women are denied the choice, and are therefore assumed to be heterosexual.

The focus group participants in McNair and Dyson's study agreed that creating a lesbian-friendly environment would assist lesbian patients. However, some participants believed that displaying lesbian health material might offend or alienate heterosexual patients, and others expressed concerns about using gender-sensitive language as it was thought that this may offend heterosexual patients.

Many large research projects still do not include sexual orientation as a research variable. The ongoing Women's Health

Australia Study (WHAS) is a study of 40000 women in three different age groups. This longitudinal study is designed to run for twenty years, with surveys every three years. The study was designed to explore factors that promote or reduce health among women who are broadly representative of the entire Australian population (Lee, 2001). A question relating to sexual orientation was included in the second survey of the young women (18–23 years) for the first time in 2000. This question was asked of the middle-aged group in survey three in 2001. A great deal of discussion and debate occurred before these questions were included in the study. Women in the older age group will not be asked this question. The justification for this omission is that heterosexual women would be offended if asked. The issue of offending heterosexual women is an interesting and disturbing one. According to much of the mainstream literature, the fear of offending heterosexual women is a valid reason for excluding lesbians. The justification of doing this is, I believe, further evidence of deep-seated homophobia. It is, in fact, another way of supporting, maintaining and reinforcing the dominant, heterosexual culture. Were this rationale to be reversed, one might justifiably ask about the lesbian who is offended and perhaps insulted every time she is assumed to be heterosexual. This situation, as my research has shown, happens repeatedly to many lesbians, particularly older lesbians. Despite the frequency of this occurrence, I have found no evidence that consideration is ever given to this situation. The right not to be offended appears to be the privilege of members of the dominant culture and certainly not of lesbians.[10] This is, in my opinion, yet another example of how the powerful group, the dominant culture (heterosexuals), have more rights than members of the powerless group (lesbians).

The issue of offending heterosexual women is more widespread than many people might be aware. Recently I had the experience of presenting findings from my study at a large

Australian health conference. I was sitting with a group of three other researchers, all from the same study, who were presenting aspects of their study to the audience. Despite each speaker being introduced by the session chair at the beginning of the session, the first speaker, before presenting her paper, made a point of reiterating that I was not part of her group and my study was in no way connected to theirs. This, I believe, was a deliberate action to distance my work on lesbians from theirs, which did not identify lesbians. Clearly, she did not want to offend or alienate heterosexual women in the audience. I believe that this was an extremely homophobic action. Fortunately, many women in the audience also interpreted this action as homophobic and several spoke to me about it afterwards.

McNair and Dyson's research demonstrated a marked lack of awareness by GPs and allied health professionals of lesbian health. The authors state that the majority of participants were not aware of the differences between lesbian health and women's health, and most viewed lesbian health as a 'subset of women's health'. From consultations with health professionals as part of my research, I found that very few health professionals believe there are any different issues for lesbians. Constantly I was asked why lesbians' experiences of menopause would be any different from heterosexual women's experiences. It is now widely recognised and understood that a person's cultural background affects her experiences with the health system, yet many health care providers are unaware that one's sexual orientation may affect the way she is seen (or not seen) and treated by health professionals within the health system.

Participants in McNair and Dyson's study expressed the view that specific articles on lesbian health would be competing with other issues that 'were of more immediate relevance' (1999, 9). Many participants stated they would read lesbian health articles if they were seeing lesbians in their practices. The issue of lesbian invisibility within primary care is obviously a barrier to health professionals' knowledge. While I was gathering information for my study, a health worker told me that the women's health service where she is employed doesn't see any lesbian clients. This is despite the fact that the service is located in the heart of a large lesbian community in an inner suburb of an Australian capital city. When I asked her how she knew that lesbians were not accessing the service, she told me, 'Well, they never say they are lesbian'. Of course, no one ever asks!

It is often suggested that having a designated lesbian health worker will improve the health system's response to lesbians. Ruth McNair and Sue Dyson suggest that the advantage of having a designated lesbian health worker available for consultation is that the doctors then have a contact point for information and referral that otherwise would not be readily available to them. While I support this view, I also see that there are some disadvantages with employing a designated lesbian health worker. One major disadvantage, I argue, is that all lesbian clients and lesbian-related issues could be redirected to this worker and as a result, other members of the health team do not increase their knowledge and awareness of lesbian health issues. Often the lesbian health worker is isolated and unsupported in the workplace and may experience homophobia from her colleagues, as well as by some consumers. This issue was highlighted by many of the lesbian health workers in my study.

Thirty-nine per cent of lesbians in my study work in health-related fields and occupations. For many of these participants, being a lesbian health worker poses additional issues related to discrimination in the workplace. Kate is employed in a rural community health centre and shared with me some of her experiences of being an out lesbian in such a workplace. I asked Kate for her thoughts on the view that it is up to lesbians to out themselves in order for positive change to occur. Her response was:

I've found myself more and more outing myself in the last . . . probably . . . four or five years. Because I felt that stopped discrimination at work and just sort of '. . . well, now you know, you can stop gossiping about me, putting me down and making homophobic jokes, and if you continue to be homophobic, coz you know directly now, because I've told you I'm a lesbian, you're in big trouble mate,' do you know what I mean? Because while they don't, there could always be that thing: 'Well, we didn't really know', and it's interesting in the workplace that I was at recently. I mean, it's really big on embracing diversity and doing all this diversity training, and I found it to be one of the most homophobic places I have ever worked in. 'Oh God, she's a lesbian', 'Oh really? But she's really nice . . .' I hate that comment. I've experienced some pretty nasty discriminative practices in workplaces over the years. At the end of the day, I guess I've started to think, what could be worse than allowing that behaviour to go on? It's so subtle, isn't it? It's like work-place bullying and stuff like that too. If you feel that something is happening people can say it's very subjective to you and yet other people might have a feeling about it. It's exclusion, not including you in conversation, and can happen in very subtle ways.

Many lesbians wrote and spoke of the homophobia and discrimination they, as well as their clients, experience in their workplaces. Leah is employed as a medical receptionist in a busy medical practice in Sydney. In an interview Leah told me how many of the sales representatives would pass homophobic comments on a variety of gay issues, for example, the Gay Games, Mardi Gras etc. Similarly she remarked, 'Doctors would commonly pass derogatory comments about patients that were openly gay and lesbian; quite demeaning remarks on their physical appearances and clothing.' [218] Leah continued to explain how her employer is of Irish Catholic descent and extremely homophobic. She has, at various times, confronted him about his attitudes; however, due to the power imbalance this is extremely difficult. Leah stated:

> I had an employer tell me that all gays and lesbians should be shot in the kneecaps. When this remark was passed, I told him to start with me if he felt so strongly. Needless to say the issue of sexuality was never brought up again. [218]

Helen, a registered nurse employed at a local community hospital, explained how she has been 'quite fortunate' with the health professionals she has dealt with. She believes this is due to the fact that she is honest and up-front with her health providers:

> I guess I have always been honest with my GP, for example, and I chose a woman GP and it turned out that she was gay. I didn't know at the time but that was OK. I guess I just be honest and people . . . well . . . you know, you just tell people how things are and it's up to them. I don't do that in a confrontational way, and if they have a problem with that, then . . . I guess I'm rather diplomatic. If I perceive there is a problem with that I let the matter rest. [1]

Although Helen has not experienced homophobia at a personal level, she is well aware of others who have been discriminated against on the basis of their sexual orientation. Helen explained about the double standard that exists, yet seems to have a philosophical approach to the issue. She commented:

> There is a double standard, too, I suppose, because sometimes people are different towards you because you are a friend. I'm aware that some of my colleagues are still of the view that if you are a lesbian you have missed out on something in your life, or you're a lesbian because of some very negative unfortunate experience with men, and it's not something they would like their daughter to be. I mean I think prejudices and things like

that just get eventually worn away like the old dripping tap analogy. You just keep on being confident and if people are going to change their view then they will. Sometimes this process happens like osmosis, you know. They suddenly realise that they don't feel quite the same, that they are more accepting than they have been in the past. I've found sometimes the attitudes of my colleagues towards lesbians who are patients has been a bit discriminatory. They've made some rather crude jokes about them but that would have to be in the minority, and on those occasions when it's happened, I've made some comment, from a professional point of view, that it's inappropriate in the first place, and secondly, if they feel that way, perhaps they shouldn't be there providing care for that person. [1]

A lesbian nurse told me how at the women's health service where she was employed, a colleague sent all workers an electronic Christmas card of a naked male. As this nurse was an out lesbian, the colleague realised that this would not be appreciated and so instead sent her an electronic card of a woman flashing her bare breasts. When the lesbian spoke to her colleague about the inappropriateness of this gesture, she was accused of not having a sense of humour and not receiving the greeting card in the thoughtful manner in which it was intended. This example highlights how the stereotype of the angry, bitter, humourless lesbian prevails and how the dominant heterosexual patriarchal culture is reaffirmed.

While pursuing my academic study, I returned to hospital nursing on a casual basis. Having not worked in midwifery for some years, I recognised the need to refresh my clinical skills and knowledge levels. I enrolled in a short breastfeeding update for midwives. This course was conducted one evening per week over a six-week period. The course facilitator is a well-known and respected lactation consultant. She has worked as a consultant for organisations including WHO[11] and UNICEF.[12]

I was enthusiastic about updating my breastfeeding knowledge, and pleased and excited to be taught by someone who is so highly regarded in this field.

During the first hour of the course, my enthusiasm and excitement turned to shock and disbelief. The course facilitator was outlining the advantages of breastfeeding and stressing the need for us, as midwives, to ensure that new mothers are made aware of the many benefits of breastfeeding. She was attempting to draw a possible link between the increasing number of childhood illnesses and conditions that are so prevalent today, such as asthma, eczema, diabetes, allergies and the large number of women who choose not to breastfeed their infants. Although I was somewhat bemused by this suggestion, with the unspoken message that 'It's all the mother's fault', it was her next jump that totally outraged me. She asked, 'Why is it that today we seem to have more homosexual people in the population than ever before?' I was wondering where this point was heading and beginning to feel most uncomfortable with this line of enquiry. As I looked around the room I observed that none of my colleagues appeared to share my sense of bewilderment at this question. Without allowing time for a response, the facilitator then suggested that the increased use of soy and other non-human milk formulas might be a contributing factor.[13] I could barely control my outrage. Still, I noticed that none of my colleagues appeared to show any signs of shock or disbelief. At that point I interjected and asked why did she regard homosexuality as a disease and what evidence did she have to support what I considered to be such an outrageous claim. From that point on, my interest level and attitude towards the course content and the facilitator changed dramatically. This real-life example highlights how many professionals have limited knowledge in the area of lesbian and gay sexual orientation and continue to impart ignorant and homophobic views. Rather than accepting that perhaps this was an outrageous claim and without any basis, the facilitator quickly turned the situation around and asked me why I had a problem with this suggestion. Attitudes such as this are extremely difficult to challenge, particularly when one is a lone voice.

In an earlier Australian report on lesbian health regarding their interactions with medical practitioners, Philomena Horsley and Sonya Tremellen were frequently told 'Lesbians don't live in our local area so I never see any' (1996, 10). This highlights the issue of lesbian invisibility and raises the concern that lesbian health issues are not regarded as legitimate concerns for heterosexual health care providers. McNair and Dyson's study revealed how 'few rural GPs would go to the bother of making their practice lesbian-friendly' (1999, 12). Lesbians, we might surmise, in the eyes of the mainstream, appear to be a bother!

A study was conducted in 1991 where 1121 US primary care doctors were surveyed to assess attitudes regarding gay and lesbian patients. Thirty-five per cent of doctors surveyed stated they would feel nervous among a group of homosexuals (Harrison, 1996, 12). The author found that in various studies:

... between 31 per cent–89 per cent of health care professionals had negative reactions to the revelation that their patients were gay or lesbian. These reactions included being embarrassed or anxious, responding in an inappropriate way, rejecting their patients directly, showing hostility and displaying excessive curiosity, pity and condescension (1996, 12).

It is these same reactions that lesbian and gay health care consumers report repeatedly in a number of more recent international and Australian studies. Such attitudes and behaviours reflect a deep-seated heterosexism and homophobia in society at large.

Carla Randall (1989) reviewed the responses of 100 American nurse educators on questions about lesbians and health care. Fifty-two per cent of the sample believed that lesbianism is 'unnatural', 34 per cent 'disgusting', 17 per cent viewed lesbianism as a disease and another 17 per cent thought that lesbians molest children. Four per cent of the nurses stated that they would refuse to care for lesbians and 13 per cent did not want a lesbian to care for them. As these are nurse educators, it is to be feared that these attitudes might be conveyed to their nursing students.

Another American survey of attitudes of 120 female nursing students demonstrated feelings of disgust and revulsion regarding lesbians (Eliason & Randall, 1991). Half of the nursing students indicated that lesbian lifestyles were unacceptable, whilst 15 per cent believed there should be laws against lesbian sexual behaviour. Twenty-six per cent of respondents said that lesbians were unacceptable and that they would avoid all contact with a lesbian. Twenty-eight per cent believed that lesbians were a high-risk group for AIDS.[14] The authors note that contact with lesbians and gay men is the most effective way of reducing homophobia and suggest that if lesbians remain 'closeted', lesbian phobia will persist.

Similarly, a survey of members of the American Gay and Lesbian Medical Association found in 1994 that '52 per cent of respondents had observed colleagues providing reduced care or denying care to patients because of their sexual orientation and 88 per cent reported hearing colleagues make disparaging remarks about lesbian, gay and bisexual patients' (Rankow, 1995, 487).

In a UK study, twenty-eight doctors were interviewed about homophobia within the medical profession (Rose, 1994). Twenty of these doctors were 'gay'[15] and eight were not. Five of the twenty-eight doctors were women, two 'non-gay' and three 'gay'. All of the gay doctors felt that homophobia exists within the medical profession, while only one 'non-gay' doctor believed that homophobia did not exist within the profession. Eleven gay doctors had not openly declared their sexual orientation due to the possible negative impact it might have on their future career. Doctors who had disclosed their sexual orientation experienced less stress than their colleagues who remained closeted. Many of the non-gay doctors claimed not to be homophobic, yet their responses to some of the interviewer's questions suggest otherwise. For example, one doctor was amazed that the study managed to attract so many gay doctors. He told the study author, 'I thought they'd be too ashamed to reply' (Rose, 1994, 586). In my mind there is no doubt that this study showed that gay doctors suffer from homophobia both outside and inside the profession.

The US National Lesbian Health Care Survey was the first large-scale publication of national data about lesbian health and health care needs. Questionnaires were completed and returned by 1925 lesbians from 50 US states. The 10-page questionnaire included the following categories: demographic information, participation in community activities and social life, 'outness', current concerns and worries, depression, anxiety and general mental health, suicide, physical and sexual abuse, anti-gay discrimination, impact of AIDS, substance use, eating disorders and counselling (Bradford et al., 1994, 229). Studies that identify lesbian health issues invariably focus on mental health, substance use and sexual and reproductive issues. It is interesting that common physical conditions are rarely included in such studies. Chronic physical conditions such as asthma, diabetes, arthritis, hypertension and epilepsy are rarely seen to be regarded as lesbian health issues, yet many lesbians, not just heterosexual women, live with these conditions. All of the conditions commonly reported to be lesbian health issues appear to be socially marginal. In other words, lesbian health issues remain marginal to other mainstream health issues.

In the US National Lesbian Health Care Survey, 88 per cent of the sample was white and the age range was between 17 and 80 years. Sixty-nine per cent had college education yet 64 per cent earned less than $20 000 per year. Compared with the US census data, the sample was younger, more educated and employed in more managerial and professional occupations than the general female population. The authors note:

> There was a distressingly high prevalence of life events and behaviors related to mental health problems. Thirty-seven per cent had been physically abused and 32 per cent had been raped or sexually attacked. Nineteen per cent had been involved in incestuous relationships while growing up. Almost one third used tobacco on a daily basis and about 30 per cent drank alcohol more than once a week; 6 per cent drank daily (1994, 239).

The authors conclude, '. . . in view of their low socio-economic status and experiences with discrimination and stigma, the capacity of lesbians in this survey to maintain interpersonal and primary relationships, educate themselves, hold responsible jobs and participate in the social, political and professional activities of their communities should be perceived as adaptive and resilient' (1994, 242). Unfortunately these types of findings often increase discrimination against lesbians as they tend to reinforce negative views and attitudes.

Access to services

Australian researchers and members of the Australian Coalition of Activist Lesbians (COAL), Helen Myers and Lavender, argue that free access to health services should be promoted through policy and practice to ensure universal availability and provision for all.

Lesbians, as a group, do not have equal access to health services. Myers and Lavender believe that groups with special needs must be identified and accorded special treatment. They suggest that lesbians have not been given 'baseline access – recognition of marginalisation and special needs'. When women from various 'target groups' are considered, they should not be assumed to be heterosexual, and when attention is given to access to services, consideration needs to be given to all of their needs. Myers and Lavender's report identifies menopause as a health issue for lesbians and suggests that although a woman's lesbianism is unlikely to affect her physiological changes, it will most likely affect the quality and delivery of her care. This finding has been well supported by the vast majority of lesbians in my menopause study. A participant explains:

> At the community centre I went to a Changing Life discussion group; the youngest woman was 42 and so we decided to focus on menopause. There was another lesbian who was very shy and closeted, and myself, among a dozen or so other women. Usually when it's relevant I'll mention I'm lesbian but there it didn't feel safe so I left the group. Where can I go to talk about my body changes and my directions without having to feel different or misunderstood because of my sexuality and emotional commitment? (quoted in Myers & Lavender, 1997, 12).

In her previously mentioned research in Victoria, Australia, Rhonda Brown found that few mainstream organisations were actually addressing the health needs and concerns of lesbians. At the end of the twentieth century, one regional women's health service, two rural community health services and a private general practice did identify lesbians as a target group and provided health care to the lesbian community in Victoria.[16] While there are many community groups offering support and information to lesbians, their work remains largely unfunded and therefore invisible. Rhonda Brown concludes that it is difficult to determine how many lesbians are accessing mainstream services, as these statistics are not routinely collected.

Patricia Stevens explains that access means more than affordable and available services and stresses that services '... are socially and culturally appropriate and geared toward effectively meeting the critical health needs of diverse communities' (1993, 40). Stevens conducted a feminist narrative study of the health care experiences of 45 lesbians from different racial/ethnic groups and on low incomes in San Francisco. Participants self-identified as lesbian, were aged between 21 and 56 years and all were English-speaking. Over half of the participants were women of colour (51 per cent) and 69 per cent of the participants had a college education. Thirty-two lesbians were interviewed individually and 13 participated in three focus groups. The findings of this study revealed that the presence and type of health care coverage determined the type of health care service available to them. Age was identified in this study as a barrier to quality health care. Sixty-four per cent of the participants had health care coverage and 36 per cent did not. According to the findings of this study, having no health care coverage was devastating. Participants without coverage spoke of health care that was so 'inadequate, dangerously inept, degrading, and victimizing that they were "driven away," becoming literal refugees from health care' (1993, 53).

Lesbians and illness

Information suggests that lesbians are not at an increased risk of illness or disease because we are lesbian. It is not one's sexual orientation that is a risk factor for illness, but the social, political and/or lifestyle factors that may have a negative impact on our health and wellbeing. Judith Bradford and Jocelyn White (2000) argue that existing studies have often lacked sufficient rigour to determine if lesbians are at an increased risk of certain health problems relevant to heterosexual women or women in general. Results from my literature searches certainly support their views.

Cancer risk

The cause of many cancers is still largely unknown and therefore accurate risk assessment is difficult and limited. Certain risk factors have been identified which place women at greater risk for certain cancers. Risk factors for many cancers increase with age or with a family history of that particular cancer. Similarly, certain lifestyle and behavioural factors can increase the risk of cancer. National and international surveys have found that lesbians may smoke and drink more alcohol, have higher body mass index, have no, or fewer, children and present for routine health screening less frequently than heterosexual women. Many of these factors place lesbians in a higher risk group for certain cancers as well as cardiovascular disease and diabetes. It has been suggested that lesbians may be at a higher risk for breast, cervical, ovarian and endometrial cancers than heterosexual women. However, as large-scale epidemiological studies have not included sexual orientation as a demographic factor to be explored, lesbians remain an invisible group of women within such studies and so pronouncements about lesbians' higher risk of ill health may be unfounded and premature.

Breast cancer

According to the Cancer Council of Victoria,[17] one in twelve Australian women will develop breast cancer at some stage in their lives, with most cases occurring after the age of 50 years. A total of 11 314 women were diagnosed with breast cancer in Australia in 2000. In that same year in Australia 2521 women died from breast cancer. In the United States it is estimated that 215 990 women will be diagnosed with breast cancer in 2004 and 40 110 women will die from breast cancer (Dibble et al., 2004, 60). In Canada it is estimated that 21 200 women will be diagnosed with breast cancer in 2004 and 5200 women will die from it (www.cbcf.org). In a similar trend, breast cancer rates are also rising in the United Kingdom. Breast cancer is the most common cancer in England and Wales. In 2000 there were almost 36000 new cases of breast cancer diagnosed. Around 11500 women died from breast cancer in England and Wales in 2000. Breast cancer is the most common cause of cancer death in women in the United Kingdom (www.statistics.gov.uk).

In a lecture to the National Gay and Lesbian Health Association, Suzanne Haynes (1994) suggested that the rate of breast cancer among lesbians might be three times higher than among heterosexual women. Although this figure has been refuted, a US study explored similarities and differences between lesbians and their heterosexual sisters in the established risks for breast cancer. The authors found that lesbians have significantly higher five-year and lifetime risk for developing breast cancer (Dibble et al., 2004). In this study, Suzanne Dibble and her team distributed anonymous surveys throughout the state of California to women 40 years and over who self-identified as lesbian. Each lesbian participant was asked to give an identical survey to her heterosexual sister (if she had one). Sisters who identified as lesbian or bisexual were not eligible to participate and they were eliminated from the analyses. The final sample consisted of 324 sister pairs.

The demographic details differed significantly between the sisters. The lesbians were slightly older, more educated, more likely to be employed full time and consequently had higher personal incomes. The investigators compared the risk estimation for developing breast cancer between the sisters and found many similarities and differences. Although there were no major differences in terms of age at onset of first period, hysterectomy rates, age at menopause and use of HRT, there were major differences in terms of pregnancy-related factors. The lesbian sisters had used oral contraceptives less, had fewer pregnancies, abortions, miscarriages and children than their straight sisters. Lesbians had a higher body mass index (BMI) than their sisters, and more lesbians exercised at least weekly. In terms of alcohol and cigarettes, more lesbians reported having a drinking problem and more lesbians than their sisters had been past smokers. These findings were supported by the WHI baseline data. A surprising finding is that more lesbians underwent breast biopsies than their heterosexual sisters. The authors are unsure if the increased number of biopsies represents actual breast changes that might indicate breast cancer or whether this shows that lesbians are aware of their increased risk of breast cancer. They suggest that this trend requires further studying (Dibble et al., 2004).

The actual incidence of breast cancer among lesbians is unknown, as cancer registries do not collect this information. A leading US gynaecologist, oncologist and surgeon, Katherine O'Hanlan claims that morbidity and mortality rates are reported to be much lower in women who have regular mammograms.[18] As my study and other studies have shown, lesbians may be less likely to perform breast self-examinations and obtain mammograms than heterosexual women (see page 84). Also, because many lesbians do not access preventative health services at the same rates as heterosexual women, they are not likely to be screened or checked regularly for early signs of breast or cervical cancers. As lesbians continue to remain invisible within the health system, it is important that further research be conducted to investigate whether or not lesbians are at a greater risk for breast and other cancers as well as to find answers to the more general questions about usefulness or distorted statistics including potential risks of mammography screening.

Ovarian and endometrial cancer

Similarly, risk factors for ovarian and endometrial cancers may be more common in lesbians than heterosexual women. Risk factors for endometrial cancer include: not having given birth (nulliparity) and obesity (Anti-Cancer Council of Victoria, 2001). It has been suggested that the use of the oral contraceptive pill may provide some protection against ovarian and endometrial cancers and the longer the pill is used, the greater the protective benefits. Although it is difficult to determine rates of contraceptive use among lesbians, it is unlikely that large numbers of lesbians would have utilised any contraceptive method extensively. Unusual uterine bleeding, referred to medically as dysfunctional uterine bleeding, might be a warning sign of endometrial cancer. This unusual or dysfunctional bleeding may occur in women after menopause, or as irregular or excessive bleeding in younger women, or in any woman, heavy bleeding that does not stop after a few days. All of these situations require investigation. However, if a woman does not have a healthy relationship with her doctor, she is unlikely to report her concerns and as a result might be putting her health at serious risk.

Cervical cancer
Few studies have been conducted regarding lesbians and cervical cancer, and as a result the incidence of cervical cancer among lesbians is not known. Doctors have often informed lesbian patients that they do not require Pap tests, as it is assumed that they do not have, or have not had in the past, sex with men. Studies suggest, however, that between 77 and 91 per cent of lesbians have had at least one prior sexual relationship with a man (Bradford et al, 1994; Bybee, 1990). This lack of knowledge by health professionals, and the perception among some lesbians that they may be less susceptible to cervical cancer than heterosexual women, means that lesbians are less likely to present for Pap tests.

Cervical cancer does appear to have a direct relationship to sexual intercourse. The most important risk factor for the development of cervical cancer is infection by the human papilloma virus (HPV) (O'Hanlan & Crum, 1996). About 30 types of HPV are spread through sexual contact, causing infection and genital warts. These types of HPV can also cause cancer of the cervix (www.4woman.gov/faq/stdhpv.htm#1). It is widely accepted that the type of HPV believed to be related to cervical cancer can be passed on to a woman by a male sexual partner during unprotected penetrative sex. What is not so clear, however, is whether this type of virus can be passed on during lesbian sex. Given this information, it is worth considering why more people are not aware of the link between heterosexual sexual activity and the development of cervical cancer. When I conducted a detailed search of the websites of a number of cancer councils and authorities, I could not find this point spelt out explicitly. It is not in the interests of mainstream society to inform women (and men) that heterosexual inter-course is a health hazard. If the vast majority of people were aware of these dangers then perhaps their sexual practices would change. It looks as if it is not in the interests of the powerful, dominant culture to inform society of the dangers associated with heterosexual sexual activity!

Marion Chinnock (1999), an Australian medical student, conducted a small qualitative study in Sydney, Australia, to identify the reasons that lesbians do or do not have Pap tests. The sample consisted of 30 women, 27 of whom identified as lesbian, aged between 20 and 49 years. The major health concerns identified by the participants included breast cancer, drug and alcohol concerns, cervical cancer, reproductive problems, health service access and doctor/patient relationship issues. Menopause as a specific health matter of concern was not mentioned.

Chinnock identified four categories involved in lesbians' decisions to present for screening or to avoid screening. These are: patient factors, doctor factors, test factors and health care factors.

Patient factors include previous negative experiences with health professionals, fear of having to answer questions concerning heterosexual sex, and a lack of awareness of cervical cancer.

Doctor factors include lack of knowledge of the need for lesbians to have Pap tests, preference for a female doctor, and a lack of lesbian-friendly doctors.

Test factors include the invasive nature of the procedure as well as the fear and embarrassment associated with the test. The main deterrent in terms of *health care factors* was the assumption of heterosexuality.

Chinnock concludes that due to the diversity of the lesbian community, targeted health promotion campaigns aimed at lesbians and Pap tests are problematic. She argues that all women with a cervix need to be aware that they are at risk of cervical cancer and thus need to be screened regardless of whether or not they have had sex with men.

Findings from Chinnock's study support those of an earlier quoted study conducted by the Australian Coalition of Activist Lesbians (Myers & Lavender, 1997). Helen Myers and Lavender identified that a lack of knowledge by health practitioners towards lesbians and cervical cancer made cervical cancer a lesbian health issue.

Mental and emotional health

The connection between lesbians and mental illness is a complex and troublesome one. Only in 1973 was homosexuality declassified as a mental illness from the *Diagnostic and Statistical Manual of Mental Disorders III* (DSM), except for those who were in conflict with their sexual orientation.[19] The DSM is a manual for diagnosing psychiatric disorders and it is widely used today by a range of mental health clinicians. In the 1990s, 42 per cent of the American Psychological Association membership still viewed homosexuality as a mental disorder. Even though homosexuality is no longer officially regarded as a mental illness, many lesbian clients have reported that heterosexual psychologists and psychiatrists still view a homosexual lifestyle as less than normal and consequently these clients seek out gay and lesbian mental health professionals.

Several of the participants in my study commented on this issue. For example:

> During a period of depression, some professionals I saw seemed to suggest a link between my mental health and my lesbianism. It was a very scary time. [6]

Presently, very little is known about the prevalence of anxiety disorders, depression, psychotic disorders and personality disorders in lesbians. The effects of societal homophobia and resulting discrimination have detrimental effects on one's self-esteem and mental health. An Australian study of 200 young lesbians reported that 60 per cent of respondents experienced feelings of depression related to their sexual orientation, 63 per cent contemplated suicide, and 30 per cent attempted suicide (Barbeler, 1992). These figures are consistent with other larger Australian and international studies.

The US National Lesbian Health Care Survey reported that lesbians experience a wide range of stress-related illness and mental health concerns. More than 50 per cent of the sample had experienced suicidal thoughts at some time, and 18 per cent had attempted suicide. One third of the women surveyed reported suffering from depression at some stage in their lives (Ryan & Bradford, 1988).

In another US study, Paul Gibson (1994) estimated that gay and lesbian youths account for 30 per cent of completed suicides annually. He suggests that gay and lesbian youth are two to three times more likely to attempt suicide as heterosexual young people. Gibson attributes the problem to living in a heterosexist society where homosexuality is stigmatised, and lesbians and gays are not acknowledged.

During consultations with Victorian lesbians, Rhonda Brown (2000) observed that the issue of mental and emotional health was raised consistently. Participants spoke of the significant stress associated with the transition from a previously heterosexual lifestyle to a lesbian lifestyle. Having to come out repeatedly to other people including health care professionals is an additional source of stress. Lesbians consulted were concerned about the lack of access to mental health services and appropriate and affordable counselling. In submissions to the Victorian Ministerial Advisory Committee on Gay and Lesbian Health (MACGLH) from members of the GLBTI[20] community and organisations, mental health issues ranked as the third most common issue raised (Brown et al., 2002, 33). Many of the submissions commented on their dissatisfaction with the quality of mental health services in Victoria and the fear of discrimination by mental health professionals with the result of reduced access to mental health services by many GLBTI people.

The Victorian Suicide Prevention Task Force identified gay, lesbian and bisexual people as a high-risk group. The report states, '. . . while comprehensive data on gay and lesbian suicide risk is limited, written and oral evidence provided to the Task Force suggests they are a particularly high-risk group, especially in rural areas' (Suicide Prevention Task Force, 1997, 40). According to this report, risk is believed to be particularly high for adolescent gays and lesbians when they acknowledge their sexual orientation and are subjected to loss of friendships, community violence and/or family rejection. The majority of studies related to suicide amongst gays and lesbians have focused on young people. Once again, older lesbians remain invisible.

Substance use

Several studies suggest that lesbians have a higher rate of drug and alcohol use than heterosexual women in the general community. Sonya Tremellen (1997) found in an Australian community survey that the percentage of lesbians smoking was 44 per cent, compared with 24.8 per cent of the general female population. Sixty-six per cent of this sample said they were unlikely to quit in the next three months, compared with 50 per cent of the general female population. Lesbians have been found to use higher amounts of alcohol for a longer period than heterosexual women (Myers & Lavender, 1997).

As part of the Women's Health Australia Study (WHAS), Lynne Hillier and colleagues (2002) conducted a sub-study that compared the licit and illicit drug using patterns of young heterosexual and non-heterosexual women in Australia. The sample comprised 9260 women aged from 22 to 27 years of whom 8409 were heterosexual and 797 non-heterosexual.[21] Findings reveal that non-heterosexual women report significantly higher usage of all types of drugs compared to heterosexual women. The use of marijuana and other illicit drugs was higher amongst the non-heterosexual women and they were significantly more likely to have injected drugs. Forty-one per cent of non-heterosexual women had used amphetamines, ecstasy and other designer drugs, compared with 10 per cent of the heterosexual women. In terms of heroin use, 7.2 per cent of non-heterosexual women reported 'lifetime experience' compared to 0.7 per cent of heterosexual women. The researchers note that young non-heterosexual women may be using drugs at higher rates than heterosexual women as a response to the effects of living in a homophobic society. These disturbing and alarming results are similar to those found in other Australian and international studies.

A study by the Australian Drug Foundation reported on alcohol and other drug use among gay, lesbian, bisexual and queer communities (GLBQ) in Victoria. Results indicate that 'Overall the alcohol and other drug use within the GLBQ sample was most commonly in the range of two-to-four-fold higher than that found in the NHS sample' (Murnane et al., 2000, 57). While the exact reasons for this high use require further research, it has been suggested that experiences of stress, history of childhood abuse and the effects of living in a homophobic world all contribute to high patterns of drug and alcohol use amongst lesbians and gay men.

Conclusion

While lesbians do not face specific health risks as a result of their sexuality, the evidence clearly suggests that the effects of heterosexism and homophobia have detrimental effects on lesbians' health and wellbeing. Due to the lack of research and the problem of homophobia it is not known if certain conditions and diseases are more common in lesbians, as presently such information is not recorded. Lesbians utilise Western medical health services less frequently than heterosexual women and some might suggest that in doing so they are putting their health at risk. On the other hand, perhaps lesbians might look towards other non-medicalised approaches in dealing with their health. Depending upon one's point of view, this non-medicalised approach might be regarded as a health-enhancing behaviour. Lesbian invisibility remains a big issue within the health care system. The lack of research on lesbian health and the failure to acknowledge lesbians as a separate group with special needs contributes to lesbian invisibility. Older lesbians remain even more under-researched. The fact that I could find only one study on lesbians and menopause is evidence of this invisibility. Clearly further empirical studies are needed. In the following chapter I discuss the unique issues that lesbians in my study face at the time of menopause.

6

'There are always different issues': Lesbians' unique experiences of menopause

Long before I began my study, I was keen to discover if there were any issues that were unique to lesbians at the time of menopause. I was also interested to learn if being a lesbian affected one's experience of menopause. Despite extensive searching, I could not find any information that looked at these issues from a lesbian perspective and so I decided to include these questions on my questionnaire. The results told me that more than half of the lesbians in my study (58 per cent) believe that that there are different issues for lesbians at this stage of life than for heterosexual women.

Although these beliefs are so common among lesbians, these issues are not acknowledged in mainstream society. In this chapter I will discuss some of the issues identified by many of the lesbians in my study that have not been documented elsewhere. The differences lesbians identified in my study relate to:
- emotional support and understanding;
- reproductive issues – loss of fertility;

- sex and sexuality (see Chapter 3);
- health services and treatment.

Emotional support and understanding

An interesting finding revealed that just under half the lesbians with partners (46 per cent) indicated that their partners were also experiencing changes related to menopause. This shared menopausal experience between partners is a phenomenon unique to lesbians. I acknowledge that every woman's experience of menopause is different, however, the fact that two women experience this transition together does give rise to a degree of support and understanding that is not present between a heterosexual woman and her male partner. Regardless of how supportive a male partner might be, he cannot experience menopause. During an interview, Pat explained to me:

> My partner and I were talking about this the other day. She's going through hers now, she's behind me because she's younger than me, and she was saying she felt good, and I felt good because I knew exactly where she was at. Even though I know everyone is an individual and they have their different experiences, she felt that I knew what . . . and I felt that I understood, as much as possible, without actually being her, but that doesn't happen with a man, because they can't. No matter how much you talk, how open you are, how comfortable you feel, it isn't the same because they can't. It is just not part of their thing at all.

Many women commented on this aspect and wrote of the level of understanding and support that this shared experience brings. Questionnaire responses include the following comments:

I think that the lesbian community would provide the atmosphere for sharing about menopause that heterosexual women may not have. Having a woman partner and lesbian friends makes it so normal to talk about it, and not only talk about it but understand from a woman's point of view. I can't imagine a heterosexual woman in menopause would get the same support and understanding from a male partner. [28]

My cycle coincides with my partner's cycle and there is greater understanding from my partner who has experienced her own symptoms. [172]

More understanding from partners and friends. No ridicule or jokes by men. [16]

I imagine it could be different in that two lesbians in a relationship going through menopause together could discuss their 'symptoms' or what they've personally noticed in more immediately empathic ways. [210]

There are two of us in the same household going through the same symptoms. It has affected our relationship. [33]

Many of the women I interviewed spoke to me about the issue of support they receive from their partner and/or lesbian friends. Anne explains:

I think we are more sensitive to each other because we go through the same process as our partner so we're more understanding of what's going on and I think we certainly discuss issues much more. I think we're certainly more alert to ourselves and we talk about it to our partners and lesbian friends. I don't think this happens to the same degree with heterosexual women, let alone with their partner and if anything, it seems like among some of my heterosexual friends that they've been really timid in wanting to even discuss it. [81]

Jill also talked about the shared experience and level of support she and her partner receive:

Well I think that one of the major things is that we both understand what the other is going through, that there is a similarity of experience that neither is going to be surprised or shocked or bothered or worried about the symptoms that the other one is experiencing. My partner and I are both meno-pausal; in fact we were in menopause when we met. Now the main symptoms are just the hot flushes, primarily, which in the night the two of us will be hot flushing simultaneously or at different times. Both of us, I mean, we are in the middle of a hot flush . . . it is quite an obvious thing and we can be flinging off bedclothes completely. It can be quite amusing, really. [58]

While many of the questionnaire responses were positive and mentioned the benefits of having a supportive female partner, other participants wrote of the loneliness and sense of isolation they experience at this time in their lives. One woman wrote:

Very little support is available to women who are openly lesbian. [164]

Similarly:

Some lesbians may not have family support during menopause, particularly those living alone. [129]

Since I've come out, I'd had no contact with my biological family so I don't know what happened in my mother's menopause. Having lesbian friends to support me and talk about the issues is a help. [45]

Another woman explained:

Being a lesbian is actually a lifelong predicament in a hetero-sexual patriarchal society. However, as a single, childless, middle-aged woman, I believe I face the same issues of isolation and hormonal discomfort as heterosexual, childless women. [21]

Other women wrote and spoke about the degree to which menopause is discussed amongst partners and lesbians friends and, as already mentioned above, some suggested that this may not be the case for some heterosexual women. Sulo explained how she and her friends talk candidly about menopause, yet notices that in her workplace and amongst her heterosexual women friends, there is more of a reluctance to discuss these issues openly and informally. In an interview, Annie commented:

When friends come around for a meal or whatever, menopause will certainly come into the conversation on a regular basis, along with retirement and lifestyle choices. It wouldn't be something that in my community of friends that we'd shy away from or feel as embarrassing, or something not to be nutted out. I think we are very open with each other about these things. For myself, it started back in consciousness-raising groups where we talked a lot about sexuality and sex, and part of the buzz of the CR era was the openness and bravery to talk about things that had never been talked about before; certainly, we had been conditioned *not* to talk about it. [131]

Leah shared with me how having a lesbian lover enables her to talk through issues that are often considered too intimate to discuss with friends or family.

I have always been able to discuss all intimate things and shadow stuff as well. I thought this was the norm until I started to discuss some of these things with my heterosexual friends and sisters. They were shocked and envious that I have been able to talk about so many things to my partner. [218]

For many lesbians in this study, the level of support and understanding gained from their partners and lesbian friends was a feature they identified as being a different issue for lesbians at the time of menopause.

Reproductive issues: Loss of fertility

The issue of loss of fertility was a common theme raised throughout many of the questionnaire and interview responses. Less than half (47.4 per cent) of the participants in my study have their own biological children, while 52.5 per cent do not. Almost 15 per cent of women in this study indicated that they co-parent a child and/or children. I did not ask if the children were the result of previous heterosexual relationships or not.

Although more than half did not have their own biological children, there was a clearly expressed view that loss of fertility was not an important issue for the majority of participants. Many lesbians explained how they rejected the notion of being past their reproductive 'use-by' date and did not view menopause as a time of loss. Several lesbians identified fertility issues as one of the major differences between lesbians and heterosexual women. If the topic of fertility was mentioned on the questionnaire, I followed it up in the interview. Some typical questionnaire comments include:

I think lesbians have a more positive attitude in that they don't see it [menopause] as an end to fertile life so much as a new stage in life. [14]

For lesbians who are childless, being past childbearing is of no consequence. Losing your attractiveness to males isn't within our reality and menopause – a sign of getting older – does not bring the same fear as hets [heterosexuals] would feel. As a feminist lesbian the experience is a positive one. [81]

Lesbians are not a homogenous group, nor are heterosexual women, but most lesbians won't have issues with changes in fertility. We could expect to have greater opportunity to discuss

any issue with our partner and other women in our community.
[67]

During the interviews, many of the participants expanded on their thoughts and explained their views in greater detail. I was totally amazed at the frankness and willingness of the women who shared with me, a total stranger, some very personal and intimate details of their lives.

Joy explained that 'bleeding and periods is about having babies'. In an interview, Joy spoke about this connection and how it did not apply to her:

From my way of thinking, bleeding and periods is about having babies, and once that whole phase of life has passed (I didn't give birth, I fostered a child) it was such a long haul, basically thirty years of bleeding. I was so glad when I stopped because I wasn't going to have a child, so I would have liked the periods to stop earlier. Yes . . . so I thought it is something to celebrate and I would have liked . . . you know how when you get the period it is a sort of celebration, so I would have liked the same sort of feeling around it, that we could have a bit of a party because I had stopped bleeding. It was so fantastic! Yes, I was a little bit excited because I had stopped. All that stuff between your legs, it was like wearing nappies once a month for thirty years! [68]

Many other lesbians I interviewed had similar ways of looking at the issue of fertility and appeared to hold common views on this topic. Nathalia told me:

I'm not at all worried about being infertile. I've never had the impulse to have children at all, even though it's true that some lesbians seem to have that impulse. There is a lot of pressure on heterosexual women to have children, and I've heard them talking about the fact that time is running out, but I've never actually had the desire to have children. It's absolutely a non-issue for me that I am becoming infertile. I don't see menopause as a transition into some negative stage of being. I guess that's partly connected to the fact that I didn't want to have children, and so I see the menstrual cycle as a bit of a waste of time and energy, because why bother if you're not going to have children? [163]

Leah had a similar opinion and explained:

For me, every single book I've picked up dealing with the change of life was obviously written by a heterosexual woman, maybe not obviously, but [it] appeared to be a heterosexual woman writing about what would happen for heterosexuality, and a lot of emphasis was put on the fact that a lot of women would start grieving because they were no longer fertile – the end of their childbearing years. Now, I find that quite interesting because I chose not to be a mother and the emphasis for me was never on childbearing. It just really has surprised me how for many heterosexual women so much emphasis was put on the end of childbearing and fertility. [218]

Anne shared these views and stated:

I know that lesbians do have children, but for a lot of us, that isn't part of what we see. Certainly for heterosexual women, childbearing is a key factor and I know many who have been distressed by getting to menopause for exactly that reason. They feel that their capacity to have children is no longer there, and even some situations where I've seen women who function in relation to their male partner, and losing their glamour looks is part of it, too. So you become at menopause this non-childbearing . . . and also this thought that you're going to become a wizened-up old prune and disintegrate physiolog-ically at the same time and you mightn't be available . . . so turned-on for sex either, so all of these things are fairly worrying. For lesbians, the pressure isn't quite the same, I don't think. We see how we relate to our partners in a different way, and it's not as a function of childbearing for the other partner as if we were in a relationship with a man, so it doesn't have the same pressure for the lesbian as it does for the heterosexual woman. It's really quite threatening for heterosexual women to be thinking that they are getting to this stage and they don't even . . . it seems a very frightening thing for them to discuss it with their partner or friends as well. [81]

Andie expanded upon this viewpoint with a feminist analysis of this issue:

Because we are all girls born into patriarchy and young women being raised in patriarchy, we are loaded with the expectation that we will bear children and that we will bear them for the sake of their fathers and for their inclusion in patriarchy. So having a child, or children, is considered natural and inevitable for women; the word 'instinctual' is sometimes used. And that is simply not true, because if it were true, if it were instinctual, every woman would be completely biologically driven to have a child, and not every one of us is, so it is not instinctual. We are not far enough along, in the women's revolution, or in having separatism for women, to have any idea at all which of us would have children and which of us wouldn't, and how many we'd have or anything else, because we never yet have had a time when it has been truly a free choice. I would imagine that in a time of real true choice that some of us would and some of us wouldn't. And that some of us might give birth but not raise a child, because her biology insisted that she do that but she wasn't, let's say, socially equipped to raise a child. Others might want to participate in raising a child, or having a child around for a period of its life, or a period of our life, but not actually birth one. And that if we were left completely to our own devices we'd probably work that out. And some of us might raise children in groups, and some of us might pair off with one, the same way we do our sex, or our work, or anything else. Also now especially, since it's a little safer in at least Western, white countries to come out as a lesbian earlier, we are able to make a little more choice as to whether to have children or not. So when it comes to menopause, the key factor for us as women is not whether we continue to have children or not. The key factor for us is, given these changes in my body, how do I function, grow, develop? Women are hurled into despair because they can't have children anymore. That is entirely a male concept of our value; it is not our idea of what makes us valuable. So menopause is supposed to be this horrible time when you lose your entire reason for being and the entire rest of your life; you're a drag on society because you are no longer childbearing. I think that lesbians can get this perspective a little quicker, because in whatever measure it is, by the very fact of being a lesbian we have removed ourselves that much from patriarchy, and that much from male domination. [7]

While Andie's articulate point of view clearly reflected the majority of lesbians' views in this study, approximately 10 per cent of lesbians in this study held opposing viewpoints. One woman commented on the questionnaire, 'Often there is grief over no children'. [221]

And two other women wrote:

Because of our 'psychological infertility', to use a current phase, I do not feel we are able to mourn the cessation of our periods. I also do not think issues surrounding decreased libido are taken seriously. [128]

Possibly less lesbians have had children and now at menopause may be a crisis of barrenness. [118]

Karla was still grieving for her child who died more than thirty years ago. During an interview, Karla shared her pain and sadness with me. At 19 years of age she had a child who died, and then at the age of 34 had a total hysterectomy. Karla described how difficult it was for her to have a hysterectomy at 34 and 'close the door on being able to have children forever'. She told me how at menopause many women are losing their own mothers, but she believes having your own children and possibly grandchildren allows 'this sense of having something to continue with'. Karla pointed out:

> To have . . . I hate to say it, but I say it in inverted commas . . . sort of 'fulfillment', you know, if you haven't got the where-withal to have children, at least you've had them and your kids have got kids and it carries on, you know . . . this sort of continuity story. Somehow that makes up for it. So being childless is very, very difficult. [156]

Sadly, Karla did not find any solace from organisations that provide support to women who have experienced stillbirths or neonatal deaths. According to Karla, most of the women attending these groups have other children and even if they don't, they are definitely not lesbians. She concluded this discussion with the following statements:

> I've never actually met – and I've met a lot of lesbians – any lesbians in my position at all, and that's very sad. That would be really good. I'm always looking for a lesbian who has lost a child and doesn't have any other children. Perhaps I should advertise in *LOTL* [laughter].[1] It's all very complex and complicated for me. [156]

At the time of interview, Karla told me that she is enjoying the company and love of her partner's adult children.

While the loss of fertility is commonly regarded in the mainstream as a problem for many women at menopause, the quotes and comments from several lesbians in my study show how this concept is often seen as irrelevant. Today many lesbians are choosing to be parents, and as a result their thoughts on fertility issues may be different when they reach menopause. For the lesbians in my study, however, having a baby, as a lesbian, was rarely considered an option.

Health services and treatment

In response to the question which asked 'are there different issues for lesbians at menopause', one of the most commonly cited differences related to health services (see Chapter 5). Many lesbians wrote on the questionnaire about difficulties they encounter when seeking medical assistance/information, such as:

I think the difference would have to do with medical assistance where the assumptions would be that the lesbian is hetero-sexual and she would be questioned on these assumptions. [28]

Yes [there are differences], only about the sex and how we deal with our pride and tell our doctor about our lifestyle, is then a problem being gay. I feel pushed aside, left out; being gay is bad to some doctors. [157]

Yes, these different issues relate to discussions between doctor/patient [about] libido problems, dry vagina etc. and the implications for sexual relationships. Lesbians have the added pressure/discomfort of correcting assumptions of hetero-sexuality and that they [doctors] are probably in a heterosexual relationship. [192]

We invariably need to talk about our partner, or the doctor asks about type of relationship, mood swings, painful intercourse, etc. [12]

Yes, there is a different kind of communication with a woman partner and different discussions with health professionals. [25]

An unexpected theme that emerged during the course of the interviews was that of repressed memories surfacing at the time of menopause. One participant shared with me her 'theory' of lowered sexual desire at the time of menopause. Andie explained how she believes that many women often experience flashbacks and vivid recollections of repressed, painful memories at the time of menopause:

> When we start menopause our system begins in effect to gear down. So here we are in pre-puberty and our hormones went like this – and then they went like this – and now [at menopause] they are going like this – . At some point we reach the pre-hormonal upsurge so in effect our endocrine system goes back to a pre-pubescent stage. We have biologically, chemical and electrical access to a state of being that we haven't had in the interim. I think that's one reason that menopausal women, especially at the very beginning of menopause, experience an increase in flashback and childhood memories. Not only memories of incest and brutalisation, but memories of what it was like to be with your own gender. [7]

Although only one lesbian mentioned this issue overtly, I decided to explore the matter in greater detail. I conducted web searches for further information on this topic but did not find any supporting data. I consulted a counsellor/advocate from a Centre Against Sexual Assault (CASA House)[2] who encouraged me to ask this question to every woman I interviewed. Annie's response to the question of repressed memories was similar to Andie's:

> Any changes in your body can bring stuff up. I think menopause makes you think about puberty, funnily enough. I was reading the book, *Woman*, by Natalie Angier, and she was talking about how at menopause your genitals start to shrink back and I suddenly thought, 'Gosh, maybe my genitals have shrunk back,' and they had and I hadn't noticed. She gives a very graphic description of how they've changed shape and go back to a kind of pre-pubescent shape. I'm talking about the labia, particularly. I just hadn't kind of checked, you know, it just happened, and then I thought about all the stuff around when I was pubescent, and you know, how extraordinary and shocking

it was that my genitals changed shape and suddenly I had these labia, and like a lot of young girls I was really worried about them; really, really worried about their size and shape and were they normal? Suddenly they're not there any more and I had a huge panic that they'd slipped away without me noticing, so that bought up lots of memories about body changes, and in the same way that at puberty things suddenly happen and . . . you know . . . you don't kind of notice them happening. And then I felt a bit sad; it was like I'd lost something. [131]

The majority of lesbians I interviewed told me how menopause/midlife was a time of reflection: reflecting upon past decisions, actions and behaviours, however, most women did not report a direct link between menopause and memories of earlier abuse and/or childhood sexual assault. Several women told me that they had dealt with matters of childhood sexual assault and other forms of abuse earlier in their lives. I asked Leah if she thought menopause was a time when repressed memories surfaced, and she replied:

It most certainly does, and I have wondered if it's because you start looking at life in a bigger sense. The complexities, the simplicities, all of these things . . . you suddenly realise there are massive contradictions and things are not as straightforward as you thought they were. I have found that I have been remembering incidents that were from my very early childhood and, thankfully having my mother here at Christmas, I was able to have a reference base to go back to. Sometimes she was quite shocked at what memories were coming up for me, especially as they were from a very young age. I am not sure why this is happening, maybe it is part of the mellowing process where the intensity of having to be so perfect, so good, etc. are being removed from us that we now have time to recall things pleasant and unpleasant. Maybe as one gets older you relax more. [218]

Elizabeth mentioned that she had done a lot of self-reflection at the age of 38 when two people close to her died suddenly:

Maybe when you have a life stage change that can happen as well but it hasn't been the case for me. Some people feel it as a sense of loss of their reproductive years, but I really do see it as a life stage, and this cycle of life that you go through. [168]

Kate explained it in the following way:

I wonder if it's just a combination of growing older and being deeply reflective, knowing that it's passed and also too often it's not unusual for a lot of women during that age period to also experience big changes in their life. Like relationship break-ups or loss of job or status or whatever it may be, which I think makes you deeply reflective because a period of your life has passed and you can never again have it back. I don't know if it's repressed memory or just allowing life experiences to come into the foreground of our lives. [44]

Merle thought that perhaps menopause/midlife might be a time where women now have time to be reflective. She remarked:

I think that perhaps it is a time when you actually do look back and maybe think about things that you haven't had time to think about before, perhaps. I think you do start to cast back, and you do start to think about your origins, maybe your family and maybe your childhood. [212]

While I do not believe that there is a biological link between repressed memories and hormones, I suggest that the issue of repressed memories at the time of midlife requires further investigation.

Another unexpected theme that surfaced early in the research process was that many women appeared to come out as lesbians around the time of menopause (see pp. 48–9). The responses, however, do reveal common themes among women who were previously married and have come out in midlife.

Participants frequently shared with me how menopause or midlife was a time where they reviewed and reflected on the 'choices' they had made in the earlier part of their lives and told me how they were now able to make different decisions. For some of the women in my study, this meant coming out as a lesbian. As Pat explained it:

So you are doing what other people expect of you and then there comes a time when you think, 'Hey, who am I really, because I can't be all things to all people that they expect me to be; now, who really am I?' I'd always been to everyone else and never been to me; you know, as the song says. I think there comes a time when most people do that. I think probably particularly women, and I think because things happen in people's lives that make them do that. I chose to work out who I am and sort it all out, and I think that you don't do that personal growth work because it's really difficult, it's hard, challenging but it's also life-changing and it's the most fantastic thing. But people don't usually do it unless something comes along in their life that makes them do it. Sometimes that's having babies, sometimes it's having a marriage breakdown, some unusual thing that makes you think, I really have to do something because I can't stand it, how it is, the way I am. Menopause might be one of those things for some women. This is just my belief and I think with me it started happening when my marriage was breaking down and I couldn't do anything about it. Because I believed that marriage was forever, whether . . . whoever you are, whatever you are, but I also believe that you have to be true to yourself and . . . do what . . . you know . . . So I was having a bit of a fight in there about knowing, yeah . . . so it caused me to do a lot of work. And so therefore I said, 'I don't like this about me because . . . I'm going to do something about changing it', and that's where that started from which happened, sort of in the middle of the time that I was having early menopause. It came by outside, something stuck up in my life where I thought I had to do something about it. From that I learnt other things, so then I thought that once the learning starts you can't ever go back. And it's a very freeing experience, so from there I sort of did other things and, yeah . . . here I am now, a lesbian. [174]

Both these quotes illustrate that lesbianism, like heterosexuality, is not biological, but rather that it is socially constructed (see Introduction). And perhaps, more importantly, both quotes explain the liberating effect of menopause – and of becoming a lesbian.

Conclusion

In this chapter I have discussed some of the general, as well as unique, issues that lesbians frequently experience at menopause, as told to me by a large group of midlife lesbians. More than half of the study participants believe there are different issues for lesbians at the time of menopause from those that exist for heterosexual women (58 per cent). These lesbian-specific issues focus on emotional support and understanding, issues relating to reproductive factors and loss of fertility, sexual issues and the experiences of homophobia and heterosexism within health services. Many of these findings have implications for health policy makers, health professionals and mainstream society. Clearly, most lesbians in this study do not experience menopause as a negative life stage and several view it with optimism and excitement.

7

Dual vision: A vision for short-term and long-term change

I would like to offer some concluding comments about my study and make some recommendations for further research. Throughout this book I have highlighted the many unique issues that lesbians experience at the time of menopause and beyond. Menopause, as discussed in the Introduction, does not occur in a vacuum and is profoundly related to social context, specifically the increasing medicalisation of women's lives. The social context in which a lesbian lives unquestionably affects every aspect of her life, and therefore needs to be considered, addressed and incorporated into understandings of her different life stages. While results from my study clearly have short-term implications for health policy makers and health care providers and require immediate attention, I believe the findings have even wider long-term ramification. The broader issues identified by participants, both in the questionnaire and interview data, raise serious concerns about midlife lesbians' wellbeing and seek long-term strategies for change.

More than twenty years ago, lesbian feminist philosopher Marilyn Frye (1983) presented a compelling argument for the continued existence of lesbian exclusion which, unfortunately, still holds true at the beginning of the twenty-first century. Frye explains that lesbians are outside of the conceptual phallo-centric[1] scheme and describes how lesbians are excluded from that scheme. She points out how a lesbian is able to see things that those belonging to the scheme cannot see. It is, according to Frye, that which she sees which is the reason for her exclusion. Frye explains:

> Lesbians are woman-seers. When one is suspected of seeing women, one is spat summarily out of reality, through the cognitive gap and into the semantic space. If you ask what became of such a woman, you may be told she became a lesbian, and if you try to find out what a lesbian is, you will be told there is no such thing. But there is. (Frye, 1983, 173)

Lesbians, particularly at menopause, as my work has shown, are definitely not seen. But they do, most definitely, exist.

In order to address the larger issues identified in my study, I have borrowed the concept of 'dual vision', or 'two sights-seeing; near and far-sightedness' from Janice Raymond (1986, 1991). In *A Passion for Friends*, Raymond explains:

> Dual vision includes, on the one hand, a keen recognition of the conditions of female existence in the man-made world. This means an acute near-sightedness that sees keenly with the ordinary faculty of sight. Realism of the world as men have fabricated it is necessary to maintain more than ordinary sight – or a feminist far-sightedness – that does not become far-flung or escapist. On the other hand, realism about the conditions of female oppression and the man-made manipulations of female existence in this world may carry us beyond hetero-relational structures, but at the same time there must be far-sighted thinking and action that suggest where we are going (1986, 207).

Dual vision enables us to see two worlds, one that focuses on the material conditions of women's lives in the here and now, and the other with a hope for a better future. The concept of near and far-sightedness, according to Janice Raymond, offers us hope. Hope allows us to realise that the present situation is not absolute and shows that alternatives actually exist. This way of seeing is, in my mind, a highly appropriate and indeed, relevant way to end this book.

Near-sightedness: Short-term vision

The focus on near-sightedness, or short-term vision, in terms of lesbians' experiences of menopause, include the following demands for positive change:

- The inclusion of midlife lesbians in all research studies. Just as gender, ethnicity and, at times class, are acknowledged and included as important variables, so too must sexual orientation be included. Funding bodies may need to list sexual orientation as a specific category in order to encourage researchers to include this variable in their research projects and submit grant proposals in this area of research.
- Lesbians, as a separate group of women, must be acknowledged in health services and in society at large. My research has illustrated the many ways in which lesbians are invisible, not only within the health services, but also in Westernised mainstream society. Cultural awareness training, in terms of sexual orientation, needs to be recognised as a priority for services working with women. Health and other workers, as well as lesbian consumers, will benefit from such training.
- Ageism is a further form of discrimination that requires special attention and discussion when connected to lesbian phobia and older women. As my study has shown, there exists an illogical view even among women's health researchers (see p. 18) that lesbians are young women. As a result of these ill-informed views, older lesbians are triply invisible within society (as women, as older women, and as lesbians).

- Findings from my study, as well as those from other published studies, confirm the need for improved practice in terms of lesbian-sensitive health care. Health services need to understand and deliver lesbian-friendly health care. This would include the creation of a 'safe' environment for a lesbian to come out, and appropriate responses when she does. Educational resources and programs that are relevant to lesbians as well as heterosexual women must be developed and applied. The assumption of across-the-board heterosexuality requires constant challenging. Services must be encouraged to examine the benefits of providing specific programs for lesbians.
- The medicalisation of menopause requires ongoing and persistent challenging. As this study has shown, many lesbians reject the notion of menopause as illness. The increasing medicalisation of a natural transition in women's lives serves to disempower and pathologise women and increase their reliance on dangerous drugs. As several participants in my study have discussed, the use of HRT (and androgens and other hormones) may be connected to concepts of sexual attractiveness and availability to men. Findings from large international studies, such as WHI (see pp. 85–7), WHIMS (pp. 92–3) and WISDOM (p. 91) illustrate the dangerous side effects associated with HRT and advise against prescribing HRT for the majority of healthy midlife women. Attention should now be paid to non-pharmaceutical agents such as strength training, weight-bearing activities, healthy eating and smoking cessation aimed at the prevention of osteoporosis and heart disease.

Recommendations for further research

My study has clearly illustrated the enormous lack of research conducted with healthy midlife lesbians in Australia and elsewhere. In order to move from a 'near-sightedness' to a 'far-sightedness', it is imperative that more research be conducted with healthy midlife lesbians. Throughout this study, I have identified numerous gaps in existing knowledge concerning different aspects of lesbian lives. I suggest that more lesbian-focussed research is needed in Australia and internationally in order to fill some of these gaps. As a result of my work, I propose that research be conducted in the following areas:

Lesbians, midlife and body image

As my research has illustrated, very few studies have been conducted with healthy middle-aged lesbians that explore the relationship between lesbians and body image. Much of the international literature includes clinical samples of young college students (see Chapter 2). Many of my study participants wrote and spoke of the importance of physical fitness in relation to questions I asked about body image. Many women commented that a lesbian and/or feminist identity provides some protection against the negative, internalised views of ageing that are frequently held by many heterosexual women. Clearly, more research is needed to explore this issue.

Lesbians and HRT use

As discussed in Chapter 4, a smaller percentage of lesbians in my study were taking HRT than was the case in other larger, published studies (see pp. 104–5). Several study participants spoke of a possible connection between the use of HRT and sexual attractiveness and/or availability to men, however, without further studies it is not possible to draw any conclusions from these comments.

The possible connection between menopause and repressed memories

One study participant spoke of her experience of menopause triggering painful repressed memories of childhood sexual assault. Following this disclosure, I asked all study participants in further interviews if they considered menopause and/or midlife to be a trigger for repressed memories. A number of participants indicated that this was a time of deep reflection and, as a consequence, several women noted that they were recalling difficult and often painful memories. I suggest that further follow-up research needs to be conducted to determine how common such experiences are.

Lesbians coming out at midlife

Many study participants remarked that they came out as lesbians just prior to menopause. A number of women spoke of the freedom that midlife brings and the accompanying sense of time for oneself. Some participants stated that menopause or midlife 'allowed' them to come out (see Chapter 6). Further studies need to discover the ages at which lesbians came out and identify the factors that assisted them in this process.

Previous heterosexual lives

While I did not ask study participants if they had been in previous long-term heterosexual relationships, several women freely shared this information with me. An interesting and unexpected finding was that two study participants (both of whom disclosed that they had been in long-term marriages) expressed extremely homophobic comments concerning lesbians, and appeared to believe negative stereotypes of lesbians (see Chapter 2). Whilst I do not wish to draw any conclusions from such a small number of comments, I believe this issue deserves further follow-up research.

Lesbians' health-seeking behaviours

As I have illustrated throughout this book, very little Australian research has been conducted on lesbians' health-seeking behaviours. Lesbians in my study were likely to have regular Pap tests for the prevention of cervical cancer, however, they were less likely to have mammography screening for the early detection of breast cancer. No explanation can be given for this inconsistency (see Chapter 5). Presently in Australia the Cancer registries do not identify a woman's sexual identity. This, I assert, is problematic. Research that explores lesbians' health-seeking behaviours and experiences of their interactions with health professionals would provide valuable data that is presently unavailable.

Even when these recommendations are implemented, I argue that this is consistent with a short-term, near-sighted vision only; a longer-term vision – far-sightedness – is needed. Indeed, there is a potential risk that these near-sighted changes may lead to mainstreaming of lesbians into 'heteroreality' (Raymond, 1986) and thus might ultimately contribute to further invisibility of lesbians.

I further suggest that language is another strategy employed by the powerful to keep lesbians invisible within mainstream society. The nature of current ideas of 'queering' lesbian existence is, I argue, highly problematic for lesbians. The use of new queer language, such as 'same-sex attracted', and pleas by the queer community to be accepted by the mainstream, are examples of this move toward further erasure of lesbians from public life.

Lesbians and the 'queer' problem

In addition to assimilating lesbians into mainstream – that is, heterosexual – culture, there is the further problem of the disappearance of lesbians into gay men's politics. Queer politics, as described by Sheila Jeffreys in *Unpacking Queer Politics* (2003), is based 'quite explicitly upon a repudiation of lesbian feminist ideas' (2003, 2). Queer politics, Jeffreys points out, wrongly assumes that lesbians and gay men are capable of forming a unified stance based upon common interests. This ignores the fact that the theory and practice of lesbian feminism resulted from the realisation that the interests of women were – and continue to be – frequently excluded in mixed political organising groups. The concept of queer, according to Jeffreys, fails to understand how patriarchy continues to oppress lesbians and aims to co-opt women to join a movement that, intentionally or not, furthers the interests of men.

As Jeffreys sees it, the actual word 'queer' is discriminatory (1994, 469). She explains how, in the past, generic words for homosexuality came to refer to men only and cites the examples of the terms 'homosexual' and 'gay' to illustrate her point. While 'queer' is regarded by its supporters as inclusive, lesbian feminists see the inclusion of such supposedly 'transgressive' or 'alternative' sexual lifestyles as problematic. Queer may include bisexuals and even heterosexuals, as long as their sexual practices are unconventional in terms of straight sexual activity (Jackson & Scott, 1996).

UK feminist Julia Parnaby claims that a queer approach is an appeal to be accepted into straight society, rather than the will to change the existing social structure (1993, 13). She writes:

> Queer is not an attempt to challenge the very basis of the hetero-patriarchal society we live in, but rather a campaign for liberal reform to increase the 'rights' of the vocal few. For lesbians to be really free from oppression it is crucial that we engage in a struggle for much more fundamental change (Parnaby, 1993, 14).

Evidence of 'queers' wanting acceptance by the dominant culture is widespread. An example is the demand by the queer community for lesbians and gays to be allowed to marry rather than questioning the institution of marriage itself. This is, I believe, an example of an appeal to be accepted into straight society. In Australia, the high-profile lesbian couple, Kerryn Phelps and Jackie Stricker, created much controversy when they married in the US in 1998. In *Kerryn & Jackie: The Shared Life of Kerryn Phelps and Jackie Stricker* (Mitchell 2002), there is an underlying theme of seeking acceptance by the dominant culture. In their biography, Phelps and Stricker want the public to see them as 'normal women' who just happen to be 'gay'. The following quote illustrates this point well:

> The filming of *Australian Story*[2] involved not just the married couple but also Kerryn's parents, her children and Jackie's parents . . . Shots of Jackie and Kerryn getting Carl and Jaime off to school in the morning like any 'normal' parents reinforced the image of them as a well-adjusted, totally integrated and supportive family. They appeared, in fact to be a gay Australian version of the Brady Bunch and Mother Knows Best all rolled into one. Everyone was smiling, happy, supportive. How could anything be wrong with how they were living their lives? They were wanting the public to understand that marriage between two women involved exactly the same feelings as heterosexual marriage. It was love and commitment, not just sex (Mitchell, 2002, 89).

However, as the findings of my study demonstrate so clearly, not all lesbians wish to be viewed as 'normal women who happen to be gay'. The views expressed by many of my study participants strongly suggest that some lesbians do not wish to be mainstreamed – that is, I argue, to become further 'invisibilised'. Many lesbians are not looking for acceptance and tolerance by the mainstream; rather they are seeking a transformation of sexual relations in our society (Auchmuty, 1996).

Sheila Jeffreys describes queer politics as 'a politics of out-siderhood' (1994, 469). She points out that queer politics accepts and celebrates the minority status of homosexuality. This stance towards homosexuality is in stark contrast to that of lesbian feminists who do not regard heterosexuality as inevitable and instead see lesbianism as a viable choice for women. Jeffreys explains:

> The lesbian feminist understanding that any woman can be a lesbian implies the rejection of minority status. It symbolises the progressive politics possible in a more hopeful time, one of opportunities for social change and brave thinking that we can only hope may re-emerge in the future. 'Queer' politics arises from a time of despair. It represents the Victorian values of the gay community (1994, 470).

The rationale for using 'queer' is often said to be that young women may not wish to identify as lesbians and feel more comfortable under the more inclusive term of 'queer'. But many lesbian feminists are highly critical of this rationale. Sheila Jeffreys reminds us that lesbians as a category do exist, and 'hundreds and thousands of women choose to live their lives within it' (Jeffreys, 2003, 159). Lesbians' unique experiences of menopause, along with other aspects of their/our lives, I decisively assert, deserve acknowledgement.

As a lesbian researcher, I am concerned that if the trend of 'queering' lesbian existence continues, how will important gaps, such as those identified in my study, be filled? If lesbians are not seen and are instead subsumed into a variety of gay men, how will knowledge about lesbians be generated and distributed? In order for lesbians to be 'seen' in ways Marilyn Frye contends they/we are not, a far-sighted vision is urgently required.

Far-sightedness: Longer-term vision

Looking through a far-sighted lens, the aim is to create a world in which heterosexuality ceases to be the norm. Far-sightedness includes living in a world beyond patriarchy, in which lesbians will be seen. This vision, not surprisingly, is one that remains difficult for most people to even imagine. The failure of past and current researchers to acknowledge sexual orientation/ identity as a variable in research studies, is evidence of the ongoing heterosexist nature of patriarchy. The fact that I could locate only two other studies concerned with lesbians and menopause is shocking proof of this invisibility. The common experience of homophobia, heterosexism, as well as ageism for the majority of lesbians in my study, highlights the need for a different way of seeing.

In a society where heteropatriarchal relations cease to be the norm, an alternative way of seeing would be possible. This society would be woman-centred, a society in which women are truly free to choose their own sexual identity and expression. I share the view of Ellen Cole and Esther Rothblum (1991), who believe that it is only when women are freed from societal pressure to live their lives, that menopause might not be the negative experience that it presently is for many women. Findings from my own study confirm the many benefits for numerous lesbian feminists who are attempting to defy heteropatriarchy and live autonomous, self-defined lives. As lesbian academic and activist Ngahuia Te Awekotuku puts it:

> Until women are free to choose, to chance, to challenge, to change, no-one is truly free. And the planet is derived of half its creative potential (1996, 58).

The voices of women in studies such as my exploration of lesbians' experiences of menopause present challenges and exciting choices. I encourage all of us to take up these challenges.

Notes

Chapter 1

1   Heterosexism is the belief that heterosexuality is the only acceptable form of sexuality.

2   Homophobia is the fear and/or hatred of lesbians and gay men.

3   As this study focused on lesbians' experiences of menopause, I believe it was essential to include the data only from women who self-identified as lesbian.

4   Eight out of the 14 women who did not wish to be interviewed are well known to me and possibly did not wish to be interviewed for this reason.

5   This number includes women who have experienced stillbirths and/or neonatal deaths.

6   The title of my thesis is 'Lesbians' Experiences of Menopause'.

7   For further information on the social construction of sexuality, see Jeffreys, 1987; Coveney et al., 1984; Kitzinger, 1987; Jackson, 1994; Jackson & Scott, 1996; Gottschalk, 2000.

8   Heteropatriarchy is a system of structures and institutions created by [heterosexual] men in order to sustain and recreate male power and female subordination (adapted from Rowland & Klein, 1996, 15).

9   In Australia, a general practitioner (GP) is a medical doctor who works in the community and treats all kinds of cases, as distinct from a consultant or medical specialist.

10   I wish to point out that menopause does not equal old age; however, menopause is a stage that usually coincides with women's midlife – apart from women who undergo premature menopause due to medical interventions such as chemotherapy and/or hysterectomies that lead to early menopause.

Chapter 2

1 See Introduction for further details.

2 Throughout this book I use the term 'Westernised' rather than 'Western' as, in addition to Europe, the US, and Canada, it allows me to include industrialised capitalist countries such as Australia and New Zealand, which are geographically located in the southern hemisphere.

3 I suggest this means 'malestream', as it reflects the views and ideals of the heterosexual male.

4 In order to protect anonymity, interviewees chose a pseudonym and for the questionnaire responses I gave them a code number, rather than using their real names.

5 I conducted a literature review on women and body image as part of my doctoral study.

6 It is worth noting that since the findings of the Women's Health Initiative study were released in 2002, HRT is now commonly referred to as Hormone Therapy (HT).

7 In an attempt to protect anonymity and confidentiality, all participants were issued with a code number. This number is used at the end of quotations cited in square brackets, e.g. [21]. Women whom I interviewed chose their own pseudonym. For this reason a combination of numbers and names are used throughout this book.

Chapter 3

1 Nett Hart (1996, 69) *From an Eroticism of Difference to an Intimacy of Equals: A Radical Feminist Lesbian Separatist Perspective on Sexuality.*

2 See: Bachmann, 1995; Dennerstein et al., 1999; Hallstrom, 1979; Leiblum et al., 1983; Sarrel, 1982; Semmens & Wagner, 1982.

3 Although Pfizer is no longer attempting to manufacture a female equivalent to Viagra, I suggest that in the near future other pharmaceutical companies will see this as a new business opportunity and will attempt to create a female version of this drug.

4 Menarche is the onset of the first menstruation.

5 Estradiol is a natural estrogenic hormone secreted chiefly by the ovaries, and is the most potent of the naturally occurring estrogens; it is used especially to treat menopausal symptoms.

6 The Jean Hailes Foundation is a leading provider of women's health services in Australia. Although located in Victoria, it is now providing women's health services nationally. Its primary focus is the health and wellbeing of the 3.3 million Australian women aged between 35 and 65.

7 GLBT refers to gay, lesbian, bisexual and transgendered.

8   Sexpo is a four-day annual event held in four major Australian cities. It is promoted by the organisers as a 'health, sexuality and lifestyle exhibition'. In Melbourne, Sexpo is sponsored by Club X – a large chain of sex shops. Over 60000 adults (40% women) visited Sexpo in Melbourne in 2002.

Chapter 4

1   In this book I use the Australian-English spelling of 'oestrogen' unless originally cited as 'estrogen'.

2   Progesterone is the name given to the female hormone that is responsible for the changes in the endometrium in the second half of the menstrual cycle preparatory for implantation, development of maternal placenta, and the development of mammary glands. In its synthetic, or human-made, form it is known as progestin or progestogen.

3   Preamble to the Constitution of the World Health Organization as adopted by the International Health Conference, New York, 19–22 June 1946; signed on 22 July 1946 by the representatives of 61 states (Official Records of the World Health Organization, no. 2, p. 100) and entered into force on 7 April 1948.

4   Alzheimer's disease is a serious disorder of the brain manifesting in premature senility.

5   Complementary therapists are highly critical of the disease model of menopause. See the resource section of this book for further references.

6   I acknowledge that some women who experience insomnia and troublesome hot flushes will request HRT in an attempt to relieve these 'symptoms'. It is not my intention to make women feel guilty for seeking out medical interventions at this time. I do, however, encourage all women to take greater control over their health and engage in open communication with their doctor about the advantages, disadvantages and suitability of such treatment. I also realise that for many lesbians, such communication may not always be easy.

7   In these studies, no experimental drug is given, however, the person's symptoms, laboratory test results, and response to treatment are observed during the course of normal medical management.

8   Since the release of the WHI findings in July 2002, the Jean Hailes Foundation has updated its information on 'Hormone Therapy Benefits and Risks'. See www.jeanhailes.org.au/issues/hrt_benefits.htm

9   BreastScreen Victoria is part of BreastScreen Australia and is jointly funded by the Victorian and Commonwealth governments. It offers free screening mammography to women over 40 years of age every two years, through a nationally-accredited service. The target group is

women aged 50–69 years, however, women over 40 years are eligible to participate.

10 If women have made a decision to take HRT and they have regular mammograms, they might want to discuss with their doctor the benefits of discontinuing HRT for two weeks prior to their mammogram.

11 Whilst these increases have been described as very small, they are, however, still increases. Women should be fully informed of the risks and benefits. I encourage women to discuss these issues openly and fully with their doctor.

12 The TGA is Australia's regulatory body for medical drugs and devices. It is a unit of the Federal Department of Health and Ageing. It carries out a range of assessment and monitoring activities to ensure therapeutic goods available in Australia are of an acceptable standard. The TGA aims to ensure that the Australian community has access, within a reasonable time, to therapeutic advances.

13 The role of the ADEC is to provide an important system of review for the evaluation work and to guide decision-making of the TGA in regard to prescription medicines.

14 This is not the first time such action has been taken.

15 Further information on the Women's Health Initiative can be obtained from the NIH website (www.nih.gov/PHTindex.htm). This website contains an enormous amount of background information and findings from these studies.

16 Medical practitioners and scientists point out that this increase is small, especially when applied to women over 65 years of age. I point out that the increases although small, are in fact increases.

17 Further attention is presently directed at what some have described as the over-prescribing of antidepressants in women. See, for example, Woodlock (2003) and McLellan (1995).

18 I am not suggesting that these healthy interventions will halt or reverse declining bone density. I am suggesting, however, that more emphasis could be placed on lifestyle factors at an earlier stage in an attempt to decrease the risk of developing such conditions.

19 Although this quote refers to ERT, I believe it is comparable to HRT. In a society such as ours that tells people their health is their own responsibility and as a result places pressure on them to adopt healthy behaviours and seek appropriate treatments, women are often pressured into taking such drugs, and they often feel it is the 'right thing' to do.

20 In this study, women were deluded by the drug companies and medical profession into thinking that hormones were the only way to prevent chronic conditions such as heart disease and Alzheimer's. As a result of

the WHI findings, such thinking amongst these groups should no longer prevail.

21   This is an erroneous view, as breast cancer can also occur outside of the breast tissue.

22   It could be argued that few lesbians would disclose their lesbian identity to an unknown interviewer over the telephone. With high levels of homophobia in the general community, many lesbians might not perceive this as a 'safe' action to take. I do not find it surprising, given the study methods, that the number of lesbians participating was extremely small.

Chapter 5

1   In order to protect anonymity, the name of the town has been omitted.

2   The options appeared in this order on the questionnaire.

3   These figures do not add up to 324. The authors do not provide any explanation for this irregularity.

4   I facilitated this group on behalf of the Victorian Department of Human Services (DHS) for the Women's Health and Wellbeing Strategy 2001. This strategy will provide a policy framework for planning, funding and delivery of services related to the health and wellbeing of Victorian women.

5   Due to the lack of an accepted definition of 'lesbian' and the effects of homophobia, which 'force' many lesbians to remain closeted, it is difficult to estimate with any degree of accuracy the number of lesbians. Ten per cent is the most widely-accepted figure (Zeidestein, 1990).

6   It must be pointed out that alternative/complementary health care providers are not always non-discriminating in their approach.

7   It is not known why lesbians in this study are more likely to have Pap tests than mammograms.

8   The high number of GPs in the study is acknowledged. Ruth McNair is a Melbourne-based GP and is heavily involved in lesbian health provision, education and research, with consumers, medical students, GPs and other health professionals.

9   This includes six nurses, one medical student, a pharmacist, a laboratory technician, a psychologist and four administrative workers.

10   See Hawthorne, 1998, for further discussion.

11   World Health Organisation.

12   United Nations Children's Fund (formerly United Nations International Children's Emergency Fund).

13   I wish to point out that this is the view of an individual lactation consultant (LC) and it is not representative of all LCs. When I have

shared this experience with other LCs they have been horrified to learn that one of their colleagues expresses these views.

14 Lesbians are not considered to be a high-risk group for AIDS. Surveys have found much lower rates of STIs among lesbians than among their heterosexual counterparts. Evidence that HIV may be transmitted between women remains inconclusive (Wilton, 1997b).

15 Rose does not use the terms 'lesbian' or 'heterosexual'. He uses only 'gay' and 'non-gay'. No explanation is given for using these terms.

16 Despite sending questionnaires and information about my study to a range of health services – including women's health services – for staff to display and/or offer to lesbian clients, I did not receive any completed questionnaires from these sources.

17 The Anti-Cancer Council of Victoria changed its name to the Cancer Council of Victoria in February 2002, to bring it in line with the names of cancer councils in other Australian states and territories.

18 Other authors and researchers disagree with these views.

19 DSM III was superseded in 1994 with the publication of DSM IV.

20 GLBTI: gay, lesbian, bisexual, transgendered and intersex.

21 Women were given five categories and asked which best described their current sexual identity. The categories are: 'exclusively heterosexual', 'mainly heterosexual', 'bisexual', 'mainly homosexual' (lesbian) or 'exclusively homosexual' (lesbian).

Chapter 6

1 *Lesbians on the Loose* (*LOTL*) is a monthly lesbian magazine published in Sydney, New South Wales, Australia. It publishes 20000 copies monthly and has a readership of 54000.

2 CASA House is a centrally located centre against sexual assault in Melbourne. It provides services to victim/survivors of sexual assault, support and consultation for friends, non-offending family members and other professionals.

Chapter 7

1 This refers to the male-centred worldview, where male characteristics are regarded as central and anything else is marginal. Lesbians, therefore, are not included in this scheme.

2 *Australian Story* is a television documentary series screened weekly on the ABC. It highlights the lives of extraordinary Australians. Dr Kerryn Phelps is a high-profile Australian lesbian, especially given her position as President of the Australian Medical Association from 2000 to 2003.

References

Adelman, Marcy (1986). *Lesbian passages: true stories told by women over 40*. Los Angeles: Alyson Publications.

American Psychiatric Association (1973). *Diagnostic and statistical manual of mental disorders* (2nd ed.). Washington, DC.

Andersson, K; Pedersen, AT; Mattsson, LA; Milsom, I (1998). Swedish gynaecologists' and general practitioners' views on the climacteric period: knowledge, attitudes and management strategies, *Acta Obstetrica et Gynecologica Scandinavica, 77*, 909–916.

Anti-Cancer Council of Victoria (2001). *Breast Cancer*. Retrieved 5 July 2001 from
http://www.accv.org.au/cancer1/patients/breast/tellmore.htm

Asher, Nancy Salkin & Asher, Kenneth Chavinson (1999). Qualitative Methods for an Outsider Looking In: Lesbian Women and Body Image. In Mary Kopala & Lisa Suzuki (Eds), *Using qualitative methods in psychology* (pp. 135–144). Thousand Oaks: Sage.

Auchmuty, Rosemary (1996). Lesbian studies: politics of lifestyle? In Lynne Harne & Elaine Miller (Eds), *All the rage: reasserting radical lesbian feminism* (pp. 200–213). London: The Women's Press.

Australasian Menopause Society (nd). *What happens at menopause – understanding menopause: a booklet of information and advice on menopause*. Glenside: Australasian Menopause Society.

Australian Institute of Health and Welfare (2000). *Australia's health 2002*. The eighth biennial report of the Australian Institute of

Health and Welfare. Canberra: Australian Government Publishing Service.

Australian Institute of Health and Welfare (2002). *Cancer in Australia 1999*. AIHW cat no. CAN 15. Canberra.

Australian Institute of Health and Welfare (nd). *National Cardiovascular Disease Database: Cardiovascular Deaths*. Retrieved 20 January 2003 from
http://www.aihw.gov.au/pls/cvd/cvd_death.show_form

Avis, Nancy E; Stellato, Rebecca; Crawford, Sybil; Johannes, Catherine; Longcope, Christopher (2000). Is there an association between menopause status and sexual functioning? sexuality, hormones and the menopausal transition. *Maturitas, 26* (2), 83–93.

Bachmann, Gloria A (1995). Influence of menopause on sexuality. *International Journal of Fertility, 40* (S1), 16–22.

Ballinger, CB (1975). Psychiatric morbidity and the menopause: screening of general population sample. *British Medical Journal, 3*, 344–346.

Ballinger, SE (1985). Psychosocial stress and symptoms of menopause: a comparative study of menopause clinic patients and non-patients. *Maturitas, 7*, 315–327.

Bancroft, J (1984). Hormones and human sexual behavior. *Journal of Sex and Marital Therapy, 10* (1), 3–21.

Banister, Elizabeth M (1999). Women's midlife experience of their changing bodies. *Qualitative Health Research, 9* (4), 520–538.

Barbeler, Vic (1992). *The young lesbian report: a study of the attitudes and behaviours of adolescent lesbians today*. Sydney: Young Lesbian Support Group, Twenty-ten Association.

Barrett-Connor, Elizabeth (1996). The menopause, hormone replacement and cardiovascular disease: the epidemiologic evidence. *Maturitas, 23*, 227–34.

Barrett-Connor, Elizabeth (1999). Sante Fe colloquium on preventive cardiovascular therapy: can coronary artery disease be stabilized or reversed? what about primary prevention? October 7–9, 1999, Sante Fe, New Mexico. Retrieved 15 May 2004 from www.acc.org/education/online/sante_fe/barrett.htm

Barry, Kathleen (1979). *Female sexual slavery*. New York: Avon Books.

Bart, Pauline B (1988). Lesbian research ethics. In Nebraska Sociological Feminist Collective (Eds), *A feminist ethic for social science research* (pp. 47–53). Lewiston, NY: Edwin Mellen Press.

Batt, Sharon (1994). *Patient no more: the politics of breast cancer*. North Melbourne: Spinifex Press.

Belchetz, Paul E (1994). Hormonal Treatment of Postmenopausal Women. *New England Journal of Medicine, 330* (15), 1062–1071.

Bell, Diane & Klein, Renate (1996). *Radically speaking: feminism reclaimed*. North Melbourne: Spinifex Press.

Berger, Gabriella E (1999). *Menopause and culture*. London: Pluto Press.

Berger, Raymond M (1984). Realities of gay and lesbian aging. *Social Work, 27,* 236–242.

Bergeron, Sherry M & Senn, Charlene Y (1998). Body image and sociocultural norms, a comparison of heterosexual and lesbian women. *Psychology of Women Quarterly, 22,* 385–401.

Bergkvist, Leif; Adami, Hans-Olov; Perssson, Ingemar; Hoover, Robert; Schairer, Catherine (1989). The risk of breast cancer after estrogen and estrogen/progestin replacement. *New England Journal of Medicine, 321* (5), 293–297.

Bhavnani, Bhagu (2002). Women's health initiative study (letter to the editor). *Journal of Obstetrics and Gynaecology Canada, 24* (9), 689–690.

Boston Women's Health Collective (1971). *Our bodies, ourselves*. New York: Simon & Schuster.

Bradford, Judith; Ryan, Caitlin & Rothblum, Esther D (1987). *The National Lesbian Health Care Survey – Final Report*. Washington DC: National Lesbian and Gay Health Foundation.

Bradford, Judith; Ryan, Caitlin & Rothblum, Esther D (1994). National lesbian health care survey: implications for mental health care. *Journal of Consulting and Clinical Psychology, 62* (2), 228–242.

Bradford, Judith & White, Jocelyn (2000). Lesbian health research. In Marlene Goldman & Maureen Hatch (Eds), *Women and health* (pp. 64–78). San Diego: Academic Press.

Bradley, Michael (2004). HRT use plummets after link to cancer. *Sydney Morning Herald*, January 8, 2004. Retrieved 1 May 2004 from www.smh.com.au

Brand, Pamela A; Rothblum, Esther D & Soloman, Laura J (1992). A comparison of lesbians, gay men and heterosexuals on weight and restricted eating. *International Journal of Eating Disorders*, *11*, 253–259.

BreastScreen Australia (2004). *Health professionals: you and BreastScreen Australia*. Australian Government Department of Health and Ageing and BreastScreen Australia. Retrieved 5 June 2004 from www.breastscreen.info.au/health_prof/index.htm

BreastScreen Queensland (nd). *Hormone replacement therapy and screening mammography. Information for general practitioners*. Queensland Government.

BreastScreen Victoria (2000). *Annual statistical report: maintaining momentum*. Carlton: BreastScreen Victoria.

British Heart Foundation (2004). *British Heart Foundation Statistics*. Retrieved 27 April 2004 from www.heartstats.org

Brogan, Maeveen (1997). Healthcare for lesbians: attitudes and experiences. *Nursing Standard*, *11* (45), 39–42.

Brown, Laura S (1987). Lesbians, weight and eating: new analyses and perspectives. In Boston Lesbian Psychologies Collective (Eds), *Lesbian psychologies: explorations and challenges* (pp. 294–309). Champaign, IL: University of Illinois Press.

Brown, Rhonda (2000). *More than lip service: the report of the Lesbian Health Information Project*. Carlton, Vic: Royal Women's Hospital.

Brown, Rhonda; Perlesz, Amaryll; Proctor, Kerry (2002). Mental health issues for GLBTI Victorians. In William Leonard (Ed.), *What's the difference? Health issues of major concern to the gay, lesbian, bisexual, transgender and intersex (GLBTI) Victorians* (pp. 29–35). Melbourne: Ministerial Advisory Committee on Gay and Lesbian Health. Victorian Government Department of Human Services.

Bybee, Deborah (1990). Michigan lesbian survey: A report to the Michigan Organization for Human Rights and the Michigan Department of Public Health. Lansing: Michigan Organization for Human Rights.

Cabot, Sandra (1995). *Menopause: hormone replacement therapy and its natural alternatives* (Rev. ed.). Paddington, NSW: Women's Health Advisory Service.

Canadian Breast Cancer Foundation (nd). Breast cancer facts. Retrieved on 1 December 2004 from http://www.cbcf.org/what/breast_cancer_facts.html

Card, Claudia (1995). *Lesbian choices*. New York: Columbia University Press.

Carroll, Nina M (1999). Optimal gynecologic and obstetric care for lesbians. *Obstetrics and Gynecology*, *93* (4), 611–613.

Cash, Thomas F & Brown, TA (1989). Gender and body images: stereotypes and realities. *Sex Roles*, *21*, 361–373.

Cash, Thomas F; Winstead, Barbara A & Janda, Louis H (1986). Body image survey report: the great American shake up. *Psychology Today*, *20*, 30–37.

Chafetz, Janet S; Sampson, Patricia; Beck, Paula & West, Joyce (1974). A study of homosexual women. *Social Work*, *19* (6), 714–723.

Chinnock, Marian (1999). Barriers to cervical screening amongst lesbian women. Paper presented at the Health in Difference 3 Conference, Adelaide, October 1999.

Chrisler, Joan C & Ghiz, Laurie (1993). Body image issues of older women. *Women and Therapy*, *14* (1/2), 67–75.

Clarke, Cheryl (1981). Lesbianism: an act of resistance. In Cherríe Moraga & Gloria Anzaldúa (Eds), *This Bridge Called My Back* (pp. 128–137). New York: Kitchen Table, Women of Color Press.

Cobleigh, MA; Berris, RF; Bush, T; Davidson, NE; Robert, NJ; Sparano, JA; Tormey, DC & Wood WC (1994). Estrogen replacement therapy in breast cancer survivors: a time for change. *Journal of the American Medical Association*, *272* (7), 540–545.

Cochran, Susan D; Mays, Vickie M; Bowen, Deborah; Gage, Suzann; Bybee, Deborah; Roberts, Susan; Goldstein, Robert S; Robison, Ann; Rankow, Elizabeth J & White, Jocelyn (2001). Cancer-related risk indicators and preventive screening behaviors among lesbians and bisexual women. *American Journal of Public Health*, *91* (4), 591–597.

Cochrane, Archibald Leman (1972). *Effectiveness and Efficiency*. London: Nutfield Provincial Hospitals Trust.

Colditz, Graham A; Hankinson, Susan E; Hunter, David J et al. (1995). The use of estrogens and progestins and the risk of breast cancer in postmenopausal women. *New England Journal of Medicine*, *332* (24), 1589–1593.

Cole, Ellen & Rothblum, Esther D (1990). Commentary on 'Sexuality and the Midlife Woman'. *Psychology of Women Quarterly*, *14*, 509–512.

Cole, Ellen & Rothblum, Esther D (1991). Lesbian sex at menopause: as good as or better than ever. In Barbara Sang, Joyce Warshow & Adrienne J Smith (Eds), *Lesbians at midlife: the creative transition* (pp. 184–193). San Francisco: Spinsters Book Company.

Coney, Sandra (1993). *The menopause industry: a guide to medicine's 'discovery' of the mid-life woman* (2nd ed.). North Melbourne: Spinifex Press.

Connors, Denise (1986). I've always had everything I wanted, but I never wanted very much: an experiential analysis of Irish-American working class women in their nineties. PhD Thesis, Brandeis University, Waltham, Massachusetts.

Cook, Judith A (1983). An interdisciplinary look at feminist methodology: ideas and practice in sociology, history and anthropology. *Humboldt Journal of Social Relations, 10,* 127–152.

Cook, Judith & Fonow, Mary Margaret (1990). Knowledge and women's interests: issues of epistemology and methodology in feminist sociological research. In Joyce McCarl Neilson, *Feminist research methods: exemplary readings in the social sciences* (pp. 69–93). Boulder, San Francisco: Westview Press.

Copper, Baba (1988). *Over the hill: reflections on ageism between women.* California: The Crossing Press.

Corea, Gena (1985). *The hidden malpractice: how American medicine mistreats women* (2nd ed.). New York: Harper & Rowe.

Corea, Gena; Klein, Renate Duelli; Hanmer, Jalna; Holmes, Helen B; Hoskins, Betty; Kishwar, Madhu; Raymond, Janice; Rowland, Robyn & Steinbacher, Roberta (1987). *Man-made women: how new reproductive technologies affect women.* Bloomington: Indiana University Press.

Coveney, Lal; Jackson, Margaret; Jeffreys, Sheila; Kay, Leslie & Mahony, Pat (1984). *The sexuality papers: male sexuality and the social control of women.* London: Hutchinson in association with The Exploration in Feminism Collective.

Crawford, Sybil L; Casey, Virginia A; Avis, Nancy E & McKinlay, Sonja M (2000). A longitudinal study of weight and the menopause transition: results from the Massachusetts Women's Health Study. *Menopause: The Journal of the North American Menopause Society, 7* (2), 96–104.

Crock, Liz; Guymer, Laurel & Klein, Renate (1999). Women's health and social control. In *Feminist perspectives on the body* (pp. 31–61). Study Guide. Geelong: Deakin University.

Crose, Royda (1999). Addressing late life developmental issues for women: body image, sexuality and intimacy. In Michael Duffy (Ed.), *Handbook of counseling and psychotherapy with older adults* (pp. 57–76). New York: John Wiley and Sons.

Cruikshank, Margaret (2003). *Learning to be old: gender, culture and aging*. Lanham, Boulder: Rowman and Littlefield.

Daly, Jeanne (1997). Facing change: women speaking about midlife. In Paul Komesaroff, Philipa Rothfield & Jeanne Daly (Eds), *Reinterpreting Menopause: Cultural and Philosophical Issues* (pp. 159–175). New York & London: Routledge.

Daly, Mary (1991). *Gyn/Ecology: the metaethics of radical feminism*. London: The Women's Press.

D'Augelli, Anthony R & Hershberger, Scott L (1993). Lesbian, gay and bisexual youth in community settings: personal challenges and mental health problems. *American Journal of Community Psychology*, 21, 421–448.

Davis, Heather A (1993). Coming of age: the experience of menopause for lesbian women. Master of Science in Nursing Thesis, MGH Institute of Health Professions, Boston.

Davis, Susan R (1998). The clinical use of androgens in female sexual disorders. *Journal of Sex and Marital Therapy*, 24, 153–163.

Davis, Susan R (2003). Testosterone: how it works, who needs it and is it safe? Media release, 19 May 2003.

Davis, Susan R (nd). Answering your patients' questions about hormone replacement therapy and alternative menopause therapies – a summary of a major review of all the published literature on HRT and alternative therapies. Distributed March 1999. Clayton, Victoria: The Jean Hailes Foundation.

Day, Anna (2002). Hormone replacement therapy – lessons from the Women's Health Initiative: primary prevention and gender health. *Canadian Medical Association Journal*, 167 (4), 361–362.

Dean, Laura; Meyer, Ilan; Robinson, Kevin et al. (2000). Lesbian, gay, bisexual and transgender health: findings and concerns. *Journal of the Gay and Lesbian Medical Association*, 4 (3), 101–151.

Deeks, Amanda Ann (1999). A biopsychosocial life-span perspective of menopause. PhD thesis, Deakin University, Geelong.

Deevey, Sharon (1990). Older lesbian women: an invisible minority. *Journal of Gerontological Nursing, 16* (5), 35–39.

Denenberg, Risa (1995). Lesbian health report. *Women's Health Issues, 5* (2), 81–91.

Dennerstein, Lorraine (1998). The controversial menopause: an overview. In Lorraine Dennerstein & Julia Shelley (Eds), *A woman's guide to menopause and hormone replacement therapy* (pp. 17–30). Washington DC: American Psychiatric Press.

Dennerstein, Lorraine; Burrows, Graham D; Wood, C & Hyman, G (1980). Hormones and sexuality: effects of oestrogen and progestogen. *Obstetrics and Gynecology, 56* (3), 316–322.

Dennerstein, Lorraine; Lehert, Philippe; Burger, Henry & Dudley, Emma (1999). Factors affecting sexual functioning of women in the mid-life years. *Climacteric, 2*, 254–262.

Dennerstein, Lorraine; Smith, Anthony MA; Morse, Carol A & Burger, Henry (1994). Sexuality and the menopause. *Journal of Psychomatic Obstetrics and Gynaecology, 15*, 59–66.

DeVault, Marjorie L (1987). Women's talk: feminist strategies for analyzing research interviews. *Women and Language, 10* (2), 33–36.

Diamant, Allison; Wold, Cheryl; Spritzer, Karen & Gelberg, Lillian (2000). Health behaviors, health status, and access to and use of health care: a population based study of lesbian, bisexual and heterosexual women. *Archives of Family Medicine, 9*, 1043–1051.

Dibble, Suzanne L; Roberts, Stephanie A & Nussey, Brenda (2004). Comparing breast cancer risk between lesbians and their heterosexual sisters. *Women's Health Issues, 14*, 60–68.

Dionne, Michelle; Davis, Caroline; Fox, John & Gurevich, Maria (1995). Feminist ideology as a predictor of body dissatisfaction in women. *Sex Roles, 33* (3/4), 277–287.

Dow, Steve (2003). Will Viagra Turn Pink? *The Age*, 20 January 2003, 4.

Doyal, Lesley (1995). *What makes women sick: gender and the political economy of health.* Houndmills, UK: Macmillan.

Doyal, Lesley (Ed.) (1998). *Women and health services: an agenda for change.* Buckingham and Philadelphia: Open University Press.

Dworkin, Sari, H (1989). Not in man's image: lesbians and the cultural oppression of body image. In Esther D Rothblum & Ellen Cole (Eds), *Loving boldly: issues facing lesbians* (pp. 27–39). New York: Harrington Park.

Dworkin, Sari H & Gutierrez, Fernando (1989). Counselors be aware: clients come in every size, shape, color and sexual orientation. *Journal of Counseling and Development, 68*, 6–10.

Eastell, R (1998). Treatment of postmenopausal osteoporosis. *New England Journal of Medicine, 338*, 736–746.

Eliason, Michelle & Randall, Carla (1991). Lesbian phobia in nursing students. *Western Journal of Nursing Research, 13*, 363–374.

Ewertz, Marianne (1996). Hormone therapy in the menopause and breast cancer risk: a review. *Maturitas, 23* (2), 239–246.

Exline, Joan L; Siegler, Irene C & Bastian, Lori A (1998). Differences in providers' beliefs about benefits and risks of hormone replacement therapy in managed care. *Journal of Women's Health, 7* (7), 879–884.

Faludi, Susan (1992). *Backlash: the undeclared war against women* (2nd ed.). London: Chatto and Windus.

Fauconnier, A; Ringa, V; Delanoe, D; Falissard, B & Breart, G (2000). Use of hormone replacement therapy: women's representations of menopause and beauty practices. *Maturitas, 35*, 215–228.

Felson, David T; Zhang, Yuqing; Hannan, Marian T et al. (1993). The effect of postmenopausal estrogen therapy on bone density in elderly women. *New England Journal of Medicine, 329* (16), 1141–1147.

Fletcher, Suzanne W & Colditz, Graham A (2002). Failure of estrogen plus progestin therapy for prevention. *Journal of the American Medical Association, 288* (3), 321–334.

Fox-Young, Stephanie; Sheehan, Mary; O'Connor, Vivienne; Cragg, Carole & Del Mar, Chris (1999). Women's knowledge about the physical and emotional changes associated with menopause. *Women & Health, 29* (2), 37–51.

Fraser, IS & Wang Y (1997). New delivery systems for hormone replacement therapy. In Barry Wren (Ed.). *Progress in the management of the menopause* (pp. 58–67). New York: Parthenon.

Friedan, Betty (1963). *The feminine mystique*. Harmondsworth: Penguin.

Frye, Marilyn (1983). *The politics of reality: essays in feminist theory*. California: The Crossing Press/Freedom.

Gambrell, R Don (1981). The role of hormones in the etiology and prevention of endometrial and breast cancer. *Acta Obstetrica et Gynecologica Scandinavica, 106* (S), 37–46.

Gannon, Linda (1998). The impact of medical and sexual politics on women's health. *Feminism and Psychology, 8* (3), 285–302.

Gannon, Linda (1999). *Women and aging: transcending the myths*. London: Routledge.

Gelfand Morris M (2000). Sexuality among older women. *Journal of Women's Health & Gender Based Medicine, 9* (S1), S15–S20.

Gentry, Susan E (1992). Caring for lesbians in a homophobic society. *Healthcare For Women International, 13* (2), 173–180.

Gettelman, Thomas E & Thompson, J Kevin (1993). Actual differences versus stereotypical perceptions of body image and eating disturbance: a comparison of male and female heterosexual and homosexual samples. *Sex Roles, 29*, 545–562.

Gibson, Paul (1994). Gay male and lesbian youth suicide. In Gary Remafedi (Ed.), *Death by denial: studies of suicide in gay and lesbian teenagers* (pp. 15–68). Boston: Alyson Publications.

Gilbert, S & Thompson, J Kevin (1996). Feminist explanations of the development of eating disorders: common themes, research findings and methodological issues. *Clinical Psychology: Science and Practice, 3*, 183–202.

Glaser, Barney G & Strauss, Anselm L (1965). *Awareness of dying*. Chicago: Aldine.

Goldman, L & Tosteson, A (1991). Uncertainty about postmenopausal estrogen: time for action not debate. *New England Journal of Medicine, 325* (11), 800–802.

Gottschalk, Hannelore Lorene (2000). Feminism and the construction of lesbianism: a comparison of lesbians' experiences in feminist and non-feminist contexts. Unpublished PhD thesis. Department of Political Science, The University of Melbourne, Parkville.

Gould, G (1998). The menopause: sexually related problems. *Nursing Standard, 12* (25), 49–56.

Grady, Deborah; Gebretsadik, T; Kerlikowske, K et al. (1995). Hormone replacement therapy and endometrial cancer risk: a meta analysis. *Obstetrics and Gynecology, 85* (2), 304–313.

Grady, Deborah; Rubin, Susan M; Petitti, Diana B et al. (1992). Hormone therapy to prevent disease and prolong life in postmenopausal women. *Annals of Internal Medicine, 117* (12), 1016–1038.

Greer, Germaine (1984). *Sex and destiny: the politics of human fertility.* London: Picador.

Greer, Germaine (1991). *The change: women, ageing and the menopause.* London: Hamish Hamilton.

Greer, Germaine (1999). *The Whole Woman.* London: Doubleday.

Griffiths, Frances & Jones, K (1995). The use of hormone replacement therapy: results of a community survey. *Family Practice, 12* (2), 163–165.

Grodstein, Francine (1996). Invited commentary: can selection bias explain the cardiovascular benefits of estrogen replacement therapy? *American Journal of Epidemiology, 143,* 979–982.

Grodstein, Francine; Stampfer, Meir J; Manson, JoAnn E et al. (1996). Post menopausal estrogen and progesterone use and the risk of cardiovascular disease. *New England Journal of Medicine, 335* (7), 453–461.

Gruskin, Elisabeth Paige (1999). *Treating lesbians and bisexual women: challenges and strategies for health professionals.* Thousand Oaks: Sage Publications.

Gupta, Madhulika, A & Schork, Nicholas, J (1993). Aging-related concerns and body image: possible future implications for eating disorders. *International Journal of Eating Disorders, 14* (4), 481–486.

Guthrie, Janet (1999). The Melbourne Women's Midlife Health Study – oral presentation to medical and nursing staff, at Family Planning Victoria. 13 March 1999.

Hall, Joanne M & Stevens, Patricia E (1991). Rigor in feminist research. *Advances in Nursing Science, 13* (3), 16–29.

Hallstrom, Tore (1977). Sexuality in the climacteric. *Clinics in Obstetrics and Gynaecology, 4* (1), 227–239.

Hallstrom, Tore & Samuelsson, Sverker (1990). Changes in women's sexual desire in middle life: the longitudinal study of women in Gothenburg. *Archives of Sexual Behaviour, 19*, 259–268.

Hammond, Charles B (1989). Estrogen replacement therapy: what the future holds. *American Journal of Obstetrics and Gynecology, 161* (6), 1864–1868.

Harding, Claudia; Knox, WF; Faragher, EB; Baildam, A & Bundred, NJ (1996). Hormone replacement therapy and tumour grade in breast cancer: prospective study in screening unit. *British Medical Journal, 312*, 1646–1647.

Harrison, Amy E (1996). Primary care of lesbian and gay patients: educating ourselves and our students. *Family Medicine, 28* (1), 10–23.

Hart, Nett (1996). From an eroticism of difference to an intimacy of equals: a radical feminist lesbian separatist perspective on sexuality. In Lilian Mohin (Ed.), *An intimacy of equals: lesbian feminist ethics* (pp. 69–77). London: Onlywomen Press.

Hart, S (1998). The relationship among body image, sexuality, and emotional distress in older women with cancer. Paper presented at the 23rd Conference of the Association for Women in Psychology, Baltimore, 5–8 March 1998.

Hawthorne, Susan (1998). Theories of power and the culture of the powerful. In *Feminist Theory, Knowledge and Power* (pp. 34–59) Study Guide. Geelong: Deakin University.

Hawthorne, Susan (2002). *Wild politics: feminism, globalisation and bio-diversity*. North Melbourne: Spinifex Press.

Hawthorne, Susan (2003a). From the lesbian body to the same-sex attracted: the depoliticising of lesbian culture. Paper presented to the Women's and Gender Studies Association Conference, University of Queensland, St. Lucia, Australia, July 2003.

Hawthorne, Susan (2003b). Lesbian Culture? Paper presented at the Feminist Fun Camp, Warrnambool, Victoria, February 2003.

Hawton, Keith; Gath, Dennis & Day Ann (1994). Sexual function in a community sample of middle-aged women with partners: effects of age, marital, socio-economic, psychiatric, gynaecological and menopausal factors. *Archives of Sexual Behavior, 23* (4), 375–395.

Haynes, Suzanne (1994). Risk of breast cancer among lesbians. Paper presented at Cancer and Cancer Risk Among Lesbians – Interactive

Working Conference. Fred Hutchinson Cancer Research Center, Seattle, Washington, December 2–4, 1994.

Heffernan, Karen (1996). Eating disorders and weight concerns among lesbians. *International Journal of Eating Disorders, 19* (2), 127–138.

Henderson, Brian E; Pagininni-Hill, Annlia & Ross, Ronald K (1991). Decreased mortality in users of estrogen replacement therapy. *Archives of Internal Medicine, 151*, 75–78.

Herzog, DB; Newman, KL; Yeh, CJ & Warshaw, M (1992). Body image satisfaction in homosexual and heterosexual women. *International Journal of Eating Disorders, 11*, 391–396.

Higgs, Joy (1997). *Qualitative research: discourse on methodologies.* Five Dock: Hampden Press.

Hillier, Lynne; McNair, Ruth; Horsley, Philomena; deVisser, Richard; Kavanagh, Anne & Pitts, Marion (2002). Substance use and emotional health issues of young lesbians and bisexual women: results from the Women's Health Australia Study. Paper presented at the Health in Difference 4 Conference, Sydney, 31 October–2 November 2002.

Hite, Shere (2003). The truth about women and sex. *The Age,* January 28, 2003, p. 11.

Horsley, P; McNair, R; Mitchell, A & Pitts, M (2001). Women's health and well-being strategy – Population group: Lesbians. Commissioned by the Department of Human Services, Victoria. pp. 1–5.

Horsley, Philomena & Tremellen, Sonya (1996). Legitimising lesbian health – challenging the 'lack of demonstrated need' argument. *Healthsharing Women, 6* (4), 8–11.

Hulley, Stephen; Grady, Deborah; Bush, Trudy et al. (1998). Randomised trial of estrogen plus progestin for secondary prevention of coronary heart disease in postmenopausal women. *Journal of the American Medical Association, 280* (7), 605–613.

Hunt, Kate (1994). A cure for all ills? constructions of the menopause and the chequered fortunes of hormone replacement therapy. In Sue Wilkinson & Celia Kitzinger (Eds), *Women and Health: Feminist Perspectives* (pp. 141–165). London: Taylor and Francis.

Hunter, Myra S (1990). Emotional wellbeing, sexual behavior and hormone replacement therapy. *Maturitas, 12*, 299–314.

Hunter, Myra S; Battersby, R; Whitehead, M (1986). Relationships between psychological symptoms, somatic complaints and menopausal status. *Maturitas, 8*, 217–228.

Hunter, Myra; O'Dea, Irene & Britten, Nicky (1997). Decision-making and hormone replacement therapy: a qualitative analysis. *Social Science Medicine, 45* (10), 1541–1548.

Hutchinson, TA; Polansky, SM & Feinstein, AR (1979). Post-menopausal oestrogens protect against fracture of the hip and distal radius: a case control study. *The Lancet, 2*, Oct 6, (8145), 705–709.

IMS Health Canada (2003). HRT prescriptions fall by nearly one third. Retrieved 1 May 2004 from www.imshealthcanada.com/htmen/1_0_13.htm

Isaacs, AJ; Britton, AR & McPherson, K (1997). Why do women doctors in the UK take hormone replacement therapy? *Journal of Epidemiology and Community Health, 51* (4), 373–377.

Jackson, Margaret (1994). *The real facts of life: feminism and the politics of sexuality*. London: Taylor and Francis.

Jackson, Stevi & Scott Sue (1996). *Feminism and sexuality: a reader*. New York: Columbia University Press.

Jacobson, Sharon (1995). Methodological issues in research on older lesbians. In Carol T Tully (Ed.), *Lesbian social services: research issues* (pp. 43–56). Haworth Press, New York.

Janelli, LM (1986). Body image in older adults: a review of the literature. *Rehabilitation Nursing, 11*, 6–8.

Jayaratne, Toby Epstein (1983). The value of quantitative methodology for feminist research. In Gloria Bowles & Renate Duelli Klein, *Theories of women's studies* (pp. 140–161). Boston: Routledge & Kegan Paul.

Jean Hailes Foundation (2002). A validation study of the female sexual satisfaction questionnaire. Retrieved on 10 June 2004 from www.jeanhailes.org.au/research/current_rp_sex.htm

Jean Hailes Foundation (2003). *Hot topics: new findings on hormone therapy. WHI hormone therapy study halted: what you need to know*. Retrieved on 10 June 2004 from http://www.jeanhailes.org.au/comment.htm

Jean Hailes Foundation (2004) Current research. Retrieved 2 May 2004 from http://www.jeanhailes.org.au/research/current.htm

Jeffreys, Sheila (Ed.) (1987). *The sexuality debates*. London: Routledge & Kegan Paul.

Jeffreys, Sheila (1993). *The lesbian heresy: a feminist perspective on the lesbian sexual revolution*. North Melbourne: Spinifex Press.

Jeffreys, Sheila (1994). The queer disappearance of lesbians. *Women's Studies International Forum*, 17 (5), 450–472.

Jeffreys, Sheila (2003). *Unpacking queer politics: a lesbian feminist perspective*. Cambridge: Polity Press.

Judd, HL (1996). The effects of HRT on endometrial histology in postmenopausal women. The Postmenopausal Estrogen/ Progestin Interventions (PEPI) Trial. *Journal of the American Medical Association*, 275 (5), 370–375.

Kaufert, Patricia (1986). Menstruation and menstrual change: women in midlife. In Virginia Olesen & Nancy Fugate Woods (Eds), *Culture, society and menstruation* (pp. 63–76). New York: Hemisphere.

Kaufert, Patricia & Gilbert, Penny (1986). Women, menopause and medicalization. *Culture, Medicine and Psychiatry*, 10 (1), 7–21.

Kavanagh, Anne M; Mitchell, Heather & Giles, Graham G (2000). Hormone replacement therapy and accuracy of mammographic screening. *The Lancet*, 355 (9200), 270–274.

Kehoe, Monika (1986). Lesbians over 65: a triply invisible minority. *Journal of Homosexuality*, 12, 139–152.

Kelly, Jennifer M (2002). Lesbians and menopause: listening to an invisibilised group in mainstream medicine. Paper presented at the Australasian Menopause Society Congress, 17 July 2002, Sydney, Australia.

Kelson, TR; Kearney-Cooke, A & Lanskey, LM (1990). Body image and body beautification among female college students. *Perception and Motor Skills*, 71, 281–289.

Kinsey, Alfred C; Pomeroy, Wardell; Martin, Clyde E & Gebhard, Paul E (1953). *Sexual behavior in the human female*. Philadelphia: WB Saunders.

Kitzinger, Celia (1987). *The social construction of lesbianism*. London: Sage Publications.

Kitzinger, Celia & Perkins, Rachel (1993). *Changing our minds: lesbian feminism and psychology.* New York and London: New York University Press.

Klein, Renate D (1983). How to do what we want to do: thoughts about feminist methodology. In Gloria Bowles and Renate Duelli Klein (Eds), *Theories of Women's Studies* (pp. 88–104). London: Routledge and Kegan Paul.

Klein, Renate (1989). *The exploitation of a desire.* Geelong: Deakin University Press.

Klein, Renate (1992). The unethics of hormone replacement therapy. *Bioethics News,* 11 (3), 24–37.

Klein, Renate (1996). Patriarchal control of women's lives: globalised fragmentation of bodies and mind. Keynote address: Violence, Abuse and Women's Citizenship International Conference, 10–15 November 1996, Brighton, UK.

Klein, Renate & Dumble, Lynette J (1994). Disempowering midlife women – the science and politics of hormone replacement therapy. *Women's Studies International Forum,* 17 (4), 327–343.

Koh, Audrey S (2000). Use of preventative health behaviors by lesbian, bisexual and heterosexual women: questionnaire survey. *Western Journal of Medicine,* 172 (6), 379–385.

Lamb, CS; Jackson, LA; Cassiday, PB & Priest, DJ (1993). Body figure preferences of men and women: a comparison of two generations. *Sex Roles,* 28 (5/6), 345–358.

Laner, Mary Riege (1997). Growing older female: heterosexual and homosexual. In Esther D Rothblum (Ed.), *Classics in lesbian studies* (pp. 87–95). New York: Harrington Park.

Laumann, Edward O; Gagnon, John H; Michael, Robert T & Michaels, Stuart (1994). *The social organisation of sexuality: sexual practices in the United States.* Chicago and London: University of Chicago Press.

Laumann, Edward; Paik, A & Rosen, R (1999). Sexual dysfunction in the united states: prevalence and predictors. *Journal of the American Medical Association,* 281, 537–544.

Lee, Christina (2001a). Lesbian invisibility within the Australian Longitudinal Study on Women's Health (personal conversation).

Lee, Christina (2001b). *Women's Health Australia: Progress on the Australian Longitudinal Study on Women's Health 1995–2000*, Brisbane: Australian Academic Press.

Leiblum, Sandra; Bachmann, Gloria; Kemmann, E; Colburn, D & Swartzman, L (1983). Vaginal atrophy in the postmenopausal woman: the importance of sexual activity and hormones. *Journal of the American Medical Association, 249* (16), 2195–2198.

Lerner, Gerda (1986). *The creation of patriarchy*. New York: Oxford University Press.

Levy, Karen (1992). *The politics of health care: medicalization as a form of social control*. Mesquite, TX: Ide House.

Lewis, Jane (1993). Feminism, the menopause and hormone replacement therapy. *Feminist Review, 43*, 38–56.

Lock, James & Steiner, Hans (1999). Gay, lesbian and bisexual youth risks for emotional, physical and social problems: results from a community-based survey. *Journal of the American Academy of Child and Adolescent Psychiatry, 38* (3), 297–304.

Lock, Margaret (1991). Contested meanings of menopause. *The Lancet, 337* (8752), 1270–1272.

Lock, Margaret; Kaufert, Patricia & Gilbert Penny (1988). Cultural construction of the menopausal syndrome: the Japanese case. *Maturitas, 10* (4), 317–332.

Ludwig, Maryanne R & Brownell, Kelly, D (1999). Lesbians, bisexual women and body image: an investigation of gender roles and social group affiliation. *International Journal of Eating Disorders, 25* (1), 89–97.

Lynch, Lee & Woods, Akia (1996). *Off the rag: lesbians writing on menopause*. Norwich, VT: New Victoria Publishers.

MacLennan, AH; Taylor, AW & Wilson, DH (1995). Changes in the use of hormone replacement therapy in South Australia. *The Medical Journal of Australia, 162*, 420–422.

MacWhannell, Doreen (1999). Taking the medical model out of menopause. *Nursing Times, 95* (41), 45–46.

Mahony, Pat & Zmroczek, Christine (1997). Why class matters. In Pat Mahony & Christine Zmroczek (Eds), *Class matters: 'working-class' women's perspectives on social class* (pp. 1–7). London: Taylor and Francis.

Malyon, AK (1982). Psychotherapeutic implications of internalised homophobia in gay men. *Journal of Homosexuality*, 7 (2/3), 59–69.

Mansfield, Phyllis Kernoff; Koch, Patricia Barthalow; Voda, Ann M (1998). Qualities midlife women desire in their sexual relationships and their changing sexual response. *Psychology of Women Quarterly*, 22, 285–303.

Mansfield, Phyllis Kernoff; Voda, Ann & Koch, Patricia Barthalow (1995). Predictors of sexual response changes in heterosexual midlife women. *Health Values*, 19 (1), 10–20.

Markowitz, L (1991). Homosexuality: are we still in the dark?' *The Family Therapy Networker*, 15 (1), 26–35.

Martin, James I & Knox, Jo (2000). Methodological and ethical issues in research on lesbians and gay men. *Social Work Research*, 24 (1), 51–60.

Mathews, W Christopher; Booth, Mary W; Turner, John D & Kessler, Lois (1986). Physicians' attitudes toward homosexuality – survey of a California county medical society. *Western Journal of Medicine*, 144 (1), 106–110.

McCoy, Norma (1998). Methodological problems in the study of sexuality and the menopause. *Maturitas*, 29, 51–60.

McGowan, Joan A & Pottern, Linda (2000). Commentary on the Women's Health Initiative. *Maturitas*, 34, 109–112.

McKie, Linda (1995). The art of surveillance or reasonable prevention? the case of cervical screening. *Sociology of Health and Illness*, 17 (4), 441–457.

McLellan, Betty (1995). *Beyond psychoppression: a feminist alternative therapy*. North Melbourne: Spinifex Press.

McNair, Ruth & Dyson, Sue (1999). Lesbian consumer visibility within primary health care – a study. Paper presented at Health in Difference 3 Conference, 21 October 1999, Adelaide.

Merriam–Webster (1993). *Collegiate Dictionary* (10th ed.). Springfield, MA: Merriam–Webster.

Miles, Matthew B & Huberman, A Michael (1994). *Qualitative data analysis: an expanded sourcebook* (2nd ed.). Thousand Oaks: Sage.

Minichiello, Victor; Aroni, Rosalie; Timewell, Eric & Alexander, Loris (1995). *In-depth interviewing: principles, techniques, analysis* (2nd ed.). Melbourne: Longman.

Mitchell, Susan (2002). *Kerryn & Jackie: the shared life of Kerryn Phelps and Jackie Stricker*. Crows Nest, Sydney: Allen & Unwin.

Moran, N (1996). Lesbian health care needs. *Canadian Family Physician*, 42, 879–884.

Morse, Carol; Smith, Anthony; Dennerstein, Lorraine; Green, Adele; Hopper, John & Burger, Henry (1994). The treatment-seeking woman at menopause. *Maturitas, 18*, 161–173.

Moynihan, Roy (2003). The making of a disease: female sexual dysfunction. *British Medical Journal, 326*, 45–47.

Murnane, Alison; Smith, Anthony; Crompton, Louise; Snow, Pamela & Munro, Geoffrey (2000). *Beyond perceptions: a report on alcohol and other drug use among gay, lesbian, bisexual and queer communities in Victoria*. Melbourne: Australian Drug Foundation.

Myers, Helen & Lavender (1997). *An overview of lesbians and health issues*. Waterloo: Coalition of Activist Lesbians Australia.

Naidoo, Jennie & Wills, Jane (2000). *Health promotion: foundations for practice* (2nd ed.). Edinburgh: Bailliere Tindall in association with the Royal College of Nursing.

National Association of Nurse Practitioners in Women's Health (2002). Hormone replacement therapy: guidance from the National Association of Nurse Practitioners. In *Women's Health Topics in Advanced Practice Nursing eJournal 2* (3), 2002. Retrieved on 27 April 2004 from www.medscape.com/viewarticle/439106

National Health and Medical Research Council (1996). Hormone replacement therapy for perimenopausal and postmenopausal women. a handbook for health professionals. Working Party, Commonwealth of Australia.

National Heart, Lung and Blood Institute (nd). What is the heart truth? Retrieved on 14 October 2004 from www.nhlbi.nih.gov/health/hearttruth/whatis/index.htm

National Institutes of Health (2002). NIH news release: NHLBI stops trial of estrogen plus progestin due to increased breast cancer risk, lack of overall benefit Retrieved on 12 March 2003 from http://www.nhlbi.nih.gov/new/press/02-07-09.htm

Northrup, Christiane (1994). *Women's bodies, women's wisdom: creating physical and emotional health and healing*. New York: Bantam Books.

Oakley, Ann (1981). Interviewing women: a contradiction in terms. In Helen Roberts, *Doing feminist research* (pp. 30–61). London: Routledge & Kegan Paul.

Oakley, Ann (1993). *Essays on women, medicine and health*. Edinburgh: Edinburgh University Press.

Oakley, Ann (1998). Science, gender and women's liberation: an argument against postmodernism. *Women's Studies International Forum, 21* (2), 133–146.

O'Brien, Mary (1981). *The politics of reproduction*. New York: Routledge & Kegan Paul.

O'Hanlan, Katherine (1995). Lesbian health and homophobia: perspectives for the treating obstetrician/gynecologist. *Current Problems in Obstetrics, Gynecology and Fertility*, July/August, 97–133.

O'Hanlan, Katherine A & Crum, Christopher P (1996). Human papillomavirus-associated cervical intraepithelial neoplasia following lesbian sex. *Obstetrics & Gynecology, 88*, pp. 702–3.

O'Neill, Sheila (1995). Presentation of menopausal problems. *Current Therapeutics*, January, 25–31.

Palacios, Santiago (1999). Current perspectives on the benefits of HRT in menopausal women. *Maturitas, 33* (S1), 1–13.

Palmer, Diane (1998). A medical perspective on menopause. In Lorraine Dennerstein & Julia Shelley (Eds), *A woman's guide to menopause and hormone replacement therapy* (pp. 43–55), Washington, DC: American Psychiatric Press.

Palmer, Diane (2002). Hormone replacement therapy: the story so far. Presentation at the Lesbian and Menopause Forum, Royal Women's Hospital, Carlton, 15 October 2002.

Pap Screen Victoria (2003). Lesbians speak out on cervical screening. Media release. Retrieved on 10 March 2003 from http://www.papscreen.org/ps/v_media/releases/030203.htm

Parnaby, Julia (1993). Queer straits. *Trouble and strife: the radical feminist magazine, 26*, Summer, 13–16.

Peterson, K Jean (1996). *Health care for lesbians and gay men: confronting homophobia and heterosexism*. New York: The Howarth Press.

Peterson, K Jean & Bricker-Jenkins, Mary (1996). Lesbians and the health care system. *Journal of Lesbian & Gay Social Services, 5* (1), 33–47.

Ramazanoglu Caroline & Holland, Janet (2002). *Feminist methodology: challenges and choices*. Thousand Oaks, London: Sage.

Randall, Carla (1989). Lesbian phobia among BSN educators. *Cassandra: Radical Nurses' Journal, 6*, 23–26.

Rankow, Elizabeth J (1995a). Lesbian health issues for the primary care provider. *Journal of Family Practice, 40* (5), 486–493.

Rankow, Elizabeth J (1995b). Breast and cervical cancer among lesbians. *Women's Health Issues, 5*, 123–129.

Rankow, Elizabeth & Tessaro, Irene (1998). Cervical cancer risk and papanicolaou screening in a sample of lesbian and bisexual women. *Journal of Family Practice, 47* (2), 139–143.

Ravnikar, VA (1987). Compliance with hormone therapy. *American Journal of Obstetrics and Gynecology, 156*, 1332–1334.

Raymond, Janice (1991). *A passion for friends: toward a philosophy of female affection*. London: The Women's Press.

Raymond, Janice (1994). *Women as wombs: reproductive technologies and the battle over women's freedom*. North Melbourne: Spinifex Press.

Rebar, RW & Spitzer, IB (1987). The physiology and measurement of hot flushes. *American Journal of Obstetrics and Gynecology, 156*, 1284–1288.

Reinharz, Shulamit (1992). *Feminist methods in social research*. New York: Oxford University Press.

Reitz, Rosetta (1977). *Menopause: a positive approach*. Radnor, PA: Chilton Book Company.

Rice, Pranee Liamputtong & Ezzy, Douglas (1999). *Qualitative research methods: a health focus*. South Melbourne: Oxford University Press.

Rich, Adrienne (1980). Compulsory heterosexuality and lesbian existence. *Signs, 5* (4), 631–660.

Riggs, Anne & Turner, Bryan S (1999). The expectation of love in older age: towards a sociology of intimacy. In Marilyn Poole & Susan Feldman (Eds), *A certain age: women growing older* (pp. 193–208). St Leonards: Allen & Unwin.

Rinzler, Carol Ann (1993). *Estrogen and breast cancer: a warning to women*. New York: Macmillan Publishing.

Robertson, M Morag (1992). Lesbians as an invisible minority in the health services arena. *Health Care for Women International, 13* (2), 155–163.

Rodin, Judith; Silberstein, Lisa & Striegel-Moore, Ruth (1985). Women and weight: a normative discontent. In TB Sonderegger (Ed.), *Nebraska symposium on motivation, psychology and gender*, 32, 267–307. Lincoln: University of Nebraska Press.

Rose, Pat (1993). Out in the open? How do nurses treat their patients and colleagues who are lesbians? *Nursing Times*, 89 (30), 50–52.

Rosser, Sue V (1993). Ignored, overlooked or subsumed: research on lesbian health and health care. *National Women's Studies Association Journal*, 5 (2), 183–203.

Rossouw, Jacques (2002). Release of the results of the estrogen plus progestin trial of the Women's Health Initiative: findings and implications. Press conference remarks, July 9, 2002 Retrieved on 10 July 2002 from
http://www.nhlbi.nih.gov/whi/hrtupd/rossouw.htm

Rothblum, Esther D (1994). Lesbians and physical appearance – which model applies? In Beverly Greene & Gregory M Herek (Eds), *Lesbian and gay psychology: theory, research, and clinical applications, psychological perspectives on lesbian and gay issues* (pp. 84–97). Thousand Oaks: Sage Publications.

Rousseau, Mary Ellen (1998). Women's midlife health – reframing menopause. *Journal of Nurse Midwifery*, 43 (3), 208–223.

Rowland, Robyn (1992). *Living laboratories*. Sydney: Pan Macmillan.

Rowland, Robyn & Klein, Renate (1996). Radical feminism: history, politics, action. In Diane Bell & Renate Klein (Eds), *Radically speaking: feminism reclaimed* (pp. 9–36). North Melbourne: Spinifex Press.

Russell, Diana EH (1990). *Rape in marriage*. Bloomington: Indiana University Press.

Ryan, Caitlin & Bradford, Judith (1988). *The national lesbian health care survey*. Washington, DC: National Lesbian and Gay Health Foundation.

Ryan, Caitlin & Bradford, Judith (1997). Lesbian Research Network: Final report – year 1. Richmond, VA: An Uncommon Legacy Foundation.

Saltman, Deborah (1994). *In transition: a guide to menopause*. Marrickville: Choice Books.

Saphira, Miriam & Glover, Marewa (1998/99). *Lesbian national health study*. New Zealand: Health Consultancy Group.

Saraga, Esther (1998). *Embodying the social: constructions of difference.* London: Routledge.

Sarrel, Philip M (1982). Sex problems after menopause: a study of fifty married couples treated in a sex counseling programme. *Maturitas,* 4, 231–237.

Sarrel, Philip (2000). Effects of hormone replacement therapy on sexual psychophysiology and behavior in postmenopause. *Journal of Women's Health and Gender-Based Medicine, 9* (S1), S25–S32.

Sarrel, Philip; Giblin, K & Liu, X (1997). Health care delivery and HRT experience: effects on HRT continuance. Presented at the semiannual meeting of the North American Menopause Society. Boston, September 1997.

Saunders, Judith M (1999). Health problems of lesbian women. *Nursing Clinics of North America, 34* (2), 381–391.

Schaad, Marie-Anne; Bonjour, Jean-Philippe & Rizzoli, Rene (2000). Evaluation of hormone replacement therapy use by the sales figures. *Maturitas, 34,* 185–191.

Schatz, Benjamin & O'Hanlan, Katherine A (1994). *Anti-gay discrimination in medicine: results of a national survey of lesbian, gay and bisexual physicians,* American Association of Physicians for Human Rights, May 1994.

Segraves, RT & Segraves, KB (1995). Human sexuality and aging. *Journal of Sex Education and Therapy, 21* (2), 88–102.

Semmens, JP & Wagner, G (1982). Estrogen deprivation and vaginal function in postmenopausal women. *Journal of the American Medical Association, 248,* 445–448.

Shelley, Julia; Smith, A; Dudley, Emma & Dennerstein, Lorraine (1995). Use of hormone replacement therapy by Melbourne women. *Australian Journal of Public Health, 1,* 387–392.

Sherwin, Susan (1992). *No longer patient: feminist ethics and health care.* Philadelphia: Temple University Press.

Shumaker, Sally A; Legault, Claudin; Rapp, Stephen R et al. (2003) Estrogen plus progestin and the incidence of dementia and mild cognitive impairment in postmenopausal women: the Women's Health Initiative Memory Study: a randomized controlled trial. *Journal of the American Medical Association, 289* (20), 2651–2662.

Siever, Michael D (1994). Sexual orientation and gender as factors in socioculturally acquired vulnerability to body dissatisfaction and eating disorders. *Journal of Consulting and Clinical Psychology, 62* (2), 252–260.

Simkin, Ruth J (1991). Lesbians face unique health care problems. *Canadian Medical Association Journal, 145* (12), 1620–1623.

Sinclair, HK; Bond, CM & Taylor, RJ (1993). Hormone replacement therapy: a study of women's knowledge and attitudes. *British Journal of General Practitioners, 43*, 365–370.

Slade, Peter David (1994). What is body image? *Behaviour Research and Therapy, 32* (5), 497–502.

Smyth, Cherry (1992). *Lesbians talk: queer notions*. London: Scarlett Press.

Solarz, Andrea L (Ed.) & Institute of Medicine (1999). *Lesbian health: current assessment and directions for the future*. Washington: National Academy Press.

Spender, Dale (1980). *Man made language*. London: Routledge & Kegan Paul.

Stagg Elliott, Victoria (2004). Estrogen-only study halted: hormone therapy promise deflates to symptom control. In *amednews.com – the newspaper for America's physicians*. Retrieved on 15 November 2004 from
http://www.ama-assn.org/amednews/2004/03/22/hll20322.htm

Stampfer, Meir J; Colditz, Graham A; Willitt, Walter C; Manson, JoAnn R; Rosner, Bernard; Speizer, Frank E et al. (1991). Postmenopausal oestrogen therapy and cardiovascular disease. Ten-year follow-up from nurses' health study. *New England Journal of Medicine, 325*, 756–762.

Stanford, JL; Weiss, NS; Voigt, LF; Daling, JR; Habel, LA & Rossing, MA (1995). Combined estrogen and progestin hormone replacement therapy in relation to risk of breast cancer in middle-aged women. *Journal of the American Medical Association, 274*, 137–143.

Stanley, Liz & Wise, Sue (1983). 'Back into the personal' or: Our attempt to construct 'feminist research'. In Gloria Bowles & Renate Duelli Klein (Eds), *Theories of women's studies* (pp. 192–209). London: Routledge & Kegan Paul.

Stevens, Claire & Tiggemann, Marika (1998). Women's body figure preferences across the life span. *Journal of Genetic Psychology, 159* (1), 94–102.

Stevens, Patricia E (1992). Lesbian health care research: a review of the literature from 1970–1990. *Health Care for Women International*, *13* (2), 91–120.

Stevens, Patricia E (1993). Marginalized women's access to health care: a feminist analysis. *Advanced Nursing Science*, *16* (2), 39–56.

Stevens, Patricia E & Hall, Joanne M (1988). Stigma, health beliefs and experiences with health care in lesbian women. *IMAGE: Journal of Nursing Scholarship*, *20* (2), 69–73.

Striegel-Moore, Ruth; Silberstein, Lisa R & Rodin, Judith (1986). Toward an understanding of the risk factors for bulimia. *American Psychologist*, *41* (3), 244–263.

Sturdee, D & Brincat, M (1988). The hot flush. In John W Studd & MI Whitehead (Eds), *The menopause* (pp. 24–42). Oxford: Blackwell Scientific Publications.

Tang, Ming-Xin & Jacobs, Diane (1996). Effect of oestrogen during menopause on risk and age at onset of Alzheimer's disease. *The Lancet*, *348* (9025), 429–432.

Te Awekotuku, Ngahuia (1996). Maori-Lesbian-Feminist-Radical. In Diane Bell & Renate Klein (Eds), *Radically speaking: feminism reclaimed* (pp. 55–61). North Melbourne: Spinifex Press.

Teede, Helena (2000). Managing menopause: exploring the choices – HRT benefits and risks. Peri-menopause, menopause and beyond. A study day for women's health nurses by Women's Health Nurse Association of Victoria, the Jean Hailes Foundation and Family Planning Victoria, 29 April 2000.

Therapeutic Goods Administration (2002). Report of Expert Committee. Convened by the Therapeutic Goods Administration to assess the findings of a report on the safety of the US Women's Health Initiative (combined hormone replacement therapy trials). Presented to the Hon. Trish Worth, Parliamentary Secretary to the Commonwealth Minister for Health and Ageing, by the Chair of the Expert Committee, Professor Martin Tattersall, 11 July 2002.

Therapeutic Goods Administration (2003a). ADEC statement on use of hormone replacement therapy: update to ADEC statement on use of hormone replacement therapy (17 October 2003). Retrieved 1 August 2004 from www.tga.health.gov.au/docs/html/hrtadec.htm

Therapeutic Goods Administration (2003b). Update to ADEC statement on use of hormone replacement therapy (17 October 2003). In *ADEC statement on use of hormone replacement therapy.* Retrieved 1 August 2004 from www.tga.health.gov.au/docs/html/hrtadec.htm

Thompson, J Kevin (1990). *Body image disturbance: assessment and treatment.* New York: Pergamon Press.

Thompson, J Kevin; Heinberg, Leslie J; Altabe, Madeline & Tantleff-Dunn, Stacey (1999). *Exacting beauty: theory, assessment and treatment of body image disturbance.* Washington, DC: American Psychological Association.

Thompson, Jan (1998). The health of lesbian women. In Cath Rogers-Clark & Angie Smith (Eds), *Women's health: a primary health care approach* (pp. 110–119). Sydney: MacLennan and Petty.

Tiefer, Lenore; Hall, Marny & Tavris, Carol (2002). Beyond dysfunction: a new view of women's sexual problems. *Journal of Sex and Marital Therapy, 28* (S), 225–232.

Tremellen, Sonya (1997). What do we need to quit? lesbians and smoking. *Healthsharing Women, 7* (3), 12–14.

Trippet, Susan E (1994). Lesbians' mental health concerns. *Health Care for Women International, 15* (4), 317–323.

University of Adelaide (2002). WISDOM ends – funding withdrawn for HRT study. Media release. Retrieved on 17 March 2003 from http://www.adelaide.edu.au/pr/media/releases/2002/wisdom ends.html

Ussher, Jane (1992). Reproductive rhetoric and the blaming of the body. In Paula Nicolson & Jane Ussher (Eds), *The psychology of women's health and health care* (pp. 31–61). Basingstoke: Macmillan Press.

Valanis, BG; Bowen, DJ; Bassford, T; Whitlock, E; Charney, P & Carter, RA (2000). Sexual orientation and health – comparisons in the women's health initiative sample. *Archives of Family Medicine, 9* (9), 843–853.

Vandenbroucke, JP (1995). How much of the cardioprotective effect of postmenopausal estrogens is real? *Epidemiology, 6* (3), 207–208.

Verghis, Sharon (2003). For the cause of a natural life: up close with Sandra Cabot. *Sydney Morning Herald,* January 25–26, 2003. p. 3.

Victorian Suicide Prevention Taskforce (1997). *Suicide prevention: Victorian taskforce report*. Melbourne: Information Victoria.

Voda, Ann, Christy, Nancy & Morgan, Julene (1991). Body composition changes in menopausal women. *Women and Therapy, 11* (2), 71–96.

Vollenhoven, Beverley (1999). The latest on hormone replacement therapy. Oral presentation to medical and nursing staff at Family Planning Victoria, 13 March 1999.

Vollenhoven, Beverley (2000). Menopause, hormone replacement therapy and alternative therapies. Printed information pack in *Perimenopause, menopause and beyond*. Melbourne: Women's Health Nurse Association of Victoria, The Jean Hailes Foundation and Family Planning Victoria.

Walling, M; Andersen, BL & Johnson, SR (1990). Hormonal replacement therapy for postmenopausal women: a review of sexual outcomes and related gynecologic effects. *Archives of Sexual Behavior, 19* (2), 119–137.

Wark, JD (1996). Osteoporotic fractures: background and prevention strategies. *Maturitas, 23*, 193–207.

Warner, Michael (1991). Fear of a queer planet. *Social Text, 9* (14), 3–17.

Webb, Dale (1999). Current approaches to gathering evidence. In Elizabeth Perkins, Ina Simnett & Linda Wright (Eds), *Evidence-based health promotion* (pp. 34–46). Chichester, New York: John Wiley and Sons.

Welch, Sarah; Collings, Sunny CD & Howden-Chapman, Phillippa (2000). Lesbians in New Zealand: their mental health and satisfaction with mental health services. *Australian and New Zealand Journal of Psychiatry. 34* (2), 256–263.

White, Jocelyn C & Dull, Valerie T (1997). Health risk factors and health seeking behavior in lesbians. *Journal of Women's Health, 6* (1), 103–112.

White, Jocelyn C & Dull, Valerie T (1998). Room for improvement: communication between lesbians and primary care providers. *Journal of Lesbian Studies, 2* (1), 95–110.

White, Jocelyn C & Levinson, Wendy (1995). Lesbians health care: what a primary care physician needs to know. *Western Journal of Medicine, 162* (5), 463–466.

Whitehead, Malcolm & Stampfer, Meir (1998). HERS – a missed opportunity. *Climacteric, 1*, 170.

Wilson, Robert A (1966). *Feminine forever*. London: W.H. Allen.

Wilton, Tamsin (1995). *Lesbian studies: setting an agenda*. New York: Routledge.

Wilton, Tamsin (1998). Gender, sexuality and healthcare: improving services. In Lesley Doyal (Ed.), *Women and health services: an agenda for change* (pp. 147–162). Buckingham: Open University Press.

Wilton, Tamsin (2000). *Sexualities in health and social care: a textbook*. Buckingham: Open University Press.

Wolf, Naomi (1991). *The beauty myth: how images of beauty are used against women*. New York: William Morrow.

Women's Health Australia (2002). *Data book for the 1998 phase 2 survey of the mid-age cohort (47–52 years). Australian Longitudinal Study on Women's Health*. The Research Centre for Gender and Health, Newcastle, Australia: University of Newcastle.

Woodlock, Delanie (2003). Marketing madness: an exploration of women and antidepressants. Unpublished honours thesis, Deakin University, Geelong.

Woodman, Natalie Jane; Tully, Carol T & Barranti, Chrystal C (1995). Research in lesbian communities: ethical dilemmas. In Carol T Tully (Ed.), *Lesbian social services: research issues* (pp. 57–66). London: Haworth Press.

Wooley, Susan C (1995). Feminist influences on the treatment of eating disorders. In Kelly Brownell & Christopher Fairburn (Eds), *Eating disorders and obesity: a comprehensive handbook*. New York: Guilford.

Worcester, Nancy & Whatley, Mariamne H (2000). More selling of HRT: still playing on the fear factor. In Nancy Worcester & Mariamne H Whatley (Eds), *Women's health: readings on social, economic and political issues* (3rd ed.) pp. 317–336. Dubuque, Iowa: Kendall Hunt Publishing.

World Health Organization (1948). Preamble to the Constitution of the World Health Organization as adopted by the International Health Conference, New York 19–22 June 1946; signed on 22 July 1946 by the representatives of 61 States (official Records of WHO, no. 2, p. 100) and entered into force on 7 April 1948. Retrieved 11 November 2002 from http://www.who.int

Wren, Barry G (1989). Management of the menopause. *Healthright, 9* (1), 35–37.

Wright, Jane (1998). Older women's experiences of the menopause. *Nursing Standard*, 12 (47), 46–48.

Writing Group for the Postmenopausal Estrogen/Progestin Intervention Trial (1995). Effects of estrogen or estrogen/progestin regimes on heart disease risk factors in postmenopausal women. *Journal of the American Medical Association*, 273, 199–208.

Writing Group for the Women's Health Initiative Investigators (2002). Risks and benefits of estrogen plus progestin in healthy postmenopausal women. Principal results from the women's health initiative randomized controlled trial. *Journal of the American Medical Association*, 288 (3), 321–333.

Young, Charlotte M; Blondin, Joan; Tensuan, Rosalinda & Fryer, Jeffrey H (1963). Body composition studies of older women, thirty-seven years of age. *Annals of the New York Academy of Sciences, 110*, 589–607.

Yusuf, Salim & Anand, Sonia (2002). Hormone replacement therapy: a time for pause. *Canadian Medical Association Journal, 167* (4), 357–359.

Zeidenstein, L (1990). Gynecological and childbearing needs of lesbians. *Journal of Nurse-Midwifery, 35* (1), 10–18.

Index

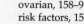